The Path to Building a Successful Nursing Career

Jennifer M. Manning

The Path to Building a Successful Nursing Career

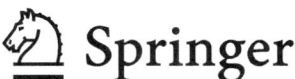 Springer

Jennifer M. Manning
Louisiana State University Health Sciences Center
School of Nursing
New Orleans, LA, USA

ISBN 978-3-030-50022-1   ISBN 978-3-030-50023-8   (eBook)
https://doi.org/10.1007/978-3-030-50023-8

This Springer imprint is published by the registered company Springer Nature Switzerland AG
The registered company address is: Gewerbestrasse 11, 6330 Cham, Switzerland

I dedicate this book to Jason, my husband of 25 years. Without your support, this book would not be possible. Thank you for supporting me on my career path. Often, you did not know why I was on my path, and you helped me anyway. Thank you for our many years together and our three beautiful children, Jason Jr., Jonathan, and Emily. Thanks for being a wonderful husband, and thank you for loving me for who I am.

Preface

Over the last 20 years, I have mentored many nurses, faculty, and nursing students. When working with nurses, I find they often need someone to layout a "path" for advancing their career. I have not found a book that addresses career advancement in this way. Many books cover elements of the path (salary, advanced practice nurse training, etc.) but do not lay it out in a comprehensive manner.

Jennifer M. Manning
New Orleans, LA, USA

Preface

I have been a registered nurse (RN) for 20 years, an advanced practice RN for 13 years, and a registered nurse educator for 12 years. My decision to become an RN did not "just happen." My journey into the nursing profession resulted from an inward journey and outward data gathering. I reflected on what I wanted in my life, assessed my strengths, obtained feedback from people in my work and personal life. I have been on a journey and feel fortunate that the path I have chosen was the right one for me. I think I have been successful in my journey, partly because I chose a path that matched what I wanted for myself and my skills.

My decision to advance my nursing career stemmed from me wanting more in my career, knowing I could make a difference, and the courage to say, "I can do this." Yes, there were people around me who doubted my path would lead to success and said: "you cannot be a mom of three children, married, work fulltime and go back to graduate school." I am so glad I did not listen to them! I now tell others to follow their dreams and not to listen to the naysayers. Keep in mind; you may be your worst enemy. Do not be afraid.

» Your future won't come to you, and you must go out and get it.

So why write this book? I worked as a director of an RN-BSN program for several years and in that time found myself meeting with RNs who achieved an associate's degree or diploma and wanted more. I felt like a broken record when I talked about the "path to building a successful nursing career." I looked for books that they could use to help guide the path and did not find one that met this specific need. I then decided I would have to write one myself. So.... to all of you out there trying to build a successful nursing career, this book is for you.

Jennifer M. Manning
New Orleans, LA, USA

Acknowledgments

This book would not be possible without all of those who have supported me in my personal and professional life. My mother and father showed me that hard work was an essential part of success. While I lost my mom far too soon in life, my dad has remained a sounding board for me and always gives me his honest opinion and encourages me to do my best in everything. My husband supported me in my career. He has been a partner in life and supported me in good times and in bad. My mentors have been invaluable to me throughout my career. Mentors led me to nursing, and mentors have led me through my many nursing roles and positions. Through their time and words of encouragement, they have shown me that success is something you can achieve and to believe in yourself.

About the Book

My book is unique in that it will address career building through the lens of the nursing profession. It is structured to begin with plotting the nursing career path. ► Chapters 1 and 2 address self-assessment, goal setting, and self-discipline. ► Chapters 3 and 4 address academic paths and non-academic paths of nursing career advancement. ► Chapter 5 addresses strategic path development, such as internal motivation, risk-taking, and work-life balance. ► Chapter 6 discusses networking, professional membership, work environments, and mentorship. ► Chapters 7 and 8 address professional growth topics such as civility, burnout, professional development, and "keeping informed." ► Chapter 9 addresses specific professionalism topics such as professional behavior, ethics, social media, and executive presence. This book will fill a gap by serving as a reference and guide for nurses interested in advancing their careers. No book gathers this information in one place specifically for the professional nurse. The work will benefit anyone interested in learning how to advance their career in nursing at any career level. The chapter topics are relevant to today's professional nurse.

Contents

III   Strategic Path Development

About the Author

Jennifer M. Manning

has 20 years of experience as a registered nurse and 12 years of advanced practice registered nurse (APRN) experience. Manning has been a nursing educator since 2007. Manning served as the Director of the RN-BSN program from 2012 to 2015 and currently serves as the Associate Dean for Undergraduate Nursing Programs. Manning is actively involved in the recruitment, progression, retention, and graduation of BSN nursing students. She has taught BSN, MSN, DNP, and research-focused doctorate nursing students. She has mentored nursing students, nursing faculty, registered nurses, and advanced practice nurses. She has authored and published approximately 20 journal publications and two book chapters. She reviews for approximately 15 journals and book publishers. She has delivered more than 50 presentations to small and large audiences at the local, statewide, and national levels. She has a variety of research interests, which aim to improve nursing education, nurse work environments, and nursing leadership.

The author currently serves as Associate Dean for Undergraduate Nursing Programs at Louisiana State University Health Sciences Center in New Orleans, LA. Dr. Manning is the registered nurse (RN) researcher at a local Magnet Hospital. She lives in Metairie, Louisiana, a suburb of New Orleans, Louisiana. She is a wife and mother of three beautiful children (Jason Jr., Jonathan, and Emily). She has a large family and extended family who she treasures greatly. She is passionate about her career in nursing and is a lifelong learner.

List of Abbreviations

AACN	American Association of Colleges of Nursing
AANP	American Association of Nurse Practitioners
ACN	Association of Camp Nursing
ACRN	Acute care registered nurse
ADN	Associate degree nurse
AG-ACNP	Adult-gerontology acute care nurse practitioner
AHRQ	Agency for Healthcare Research and Quality
ANA	American Nurses Association
ANCC	American Nurses Credential Center
AONL	American Organization for Nursing Leadership
APRN	Advanced practice registered nurse
BLS	Bureau of Labor Statistics
CCM	Certified case manager
CCRN	Critical care registered nurse
CE	Continuing education
CNA	Certified nursing assistant
CNL	Clinical nurse leader
CNM	Certified nurse midwife
CNS	Clinical nurse specialist
COHN	Certified occupational health nurse
CPHQ	Certified professional in healthcare quality
CRNA	Certified registered nurse anesthetists
EI	Emotional intelligence
HWE	Healthy work environment
HWNC-BC	Health and Wellness Nurse Coach Board Certified
ICN	International Council of Nurses
LACE	Licensure, accreditation, certification, and education
LNC	Legal nurse consultant
LPN	Licensed practical nurse
NCSBN	National Councils for State Boards of Nursing
NDNQI	National Database of Nursing Quality Indicators
NINR	National Institute of Nursing Research
NNP	Neonatal nurse practitioner
NP	Nurse practitioner

NSNA	National Student Nurses Association
PHN	Public health nurse
RN	Registered nurse
RN-BC	Registered nurse board certified
SMART	Specific, measurable, achievable, relevant, time-bound

Plotting Your Career Path

Plotting your career path is a purposeful and intentional process. One's career consists of a combination of their work and personal life. A career includes various roles, places, and circumstances encountered in a lifetime. A career can be thought of as a life career development and is a life process. A job is only one part of a career and does not wholly represent the career-building process. When one views their career from a broad perspective, there is a clearer understanding of the concept and the scope from a career development perspective.

As a life process, career development is ongoing and goes through various phases. I often think of these phases as "chapters." Some chapters may include more growth than others. In the growth chapters, a person strives to accomplish tasks that correspond to the various roles in their career. Some chapters tell the story of personal struggles we must all face. Some chapters tell the story of personal and professional growth where we go beyond our current stage in life and develop.

Career development is a process that undergoes transition and change. A person is gathering information for the next as they navigate through their development. This transitional process begins with a "looking inward."

Contents

Self-Assessment

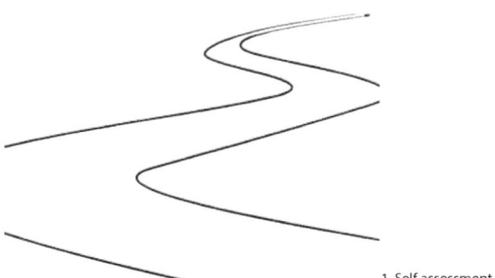

1. Self assessment

Contents

© Springer Nature Switzerland AG 2020
J. M. Manning, *The Path to Building a Successful Nursing Career*,
https://doi.org/10.1007/978-3-030-50023-8_1

Can you learn to be a mirror for yourself?

1

1.1 Introduction

Conducting a self-assessment is essential in gaining insight into one's values, skill sets, strengths, and weaknesses. Through a self-assessment, one can begin to understand their values and beliefs. They can understand what skills they possess. From there, one's vision develops. One can identify their strengths and weaknesses. By bringing this information to the forefront of one's thinking, a person can make better decisions when chartering a career path. A clear self-assessment can assist in correcting areas in one's life, which seems "off path" or just does not "feel right."

The first step in plotting a successful and rewarding career path should begin with a self-assessment. A self-assessment includes learning about oneself so that a career trajectory can be selected, which is the best fit for you. The purpose of a self-assessment provides some direction about the type of career you should consider pursuing. A self-assessment is a data-gathering and evaluation process where work-related values, beliefs, skills, vision, strengths, and weaknesses are evaluated.

The best way to begin a self-assessment is through a formal approach. Many tools exist to assist with completing a formal self-assessment. When conducting a self-assessment, it is crucial to reflect. A self-assessment requires time, honesty with yourself, and writing reflective thoughts. It is also essential to ask for feedback from others about your reflection as you develop a plan to move forward on your career path based on the insights you obtain.

1.2 Values

The definition of "values" is the ideas and beliefs which are of importance to you (Merriam-Webster's 1999). Examples of values may include job security, autonomy, prestige, flexible work schedules, leisure time, or high salary. Understanding which values are of importance to you and ensuring your values are supported in your future career can lead to high-level job satisfaction and further career development. Values are typically stable for most people. They do not have strict boundaries. As you grow and develop, your values may change somewhat. For example, income may be a priority in your life at some point in your career; work–life balance may be a priority at another point in your career. Values change over time because you, as a person, grow and develop. For example, if you marry and/or have children, the belief regarding what is important to you changes. Keeping in touch with your values is key to building a successful nursing career.

When the things you do in your life, such as your career and hobbies, match your values and beliefs, you are often satisfied with your life. When your career and hobbies do not match, life may feel "off" or like something is "wrong," eventually leading to unhappiness. When you understand your values, you can make the right decisions to some of the essential questions in your life. For example, you may be wondering where to go in life. Understanding your values can help you evaluate and decide if you should stay in this job, should I accept this promotion, should I follow tradition or start a new path in my life?

Case Example 1.1 Sample Questions to Ask When Exploring Personal Values

Consider the following questions. Using a journal, write the answer to the following questions:

Step 1:

(a) Think of a happy time in your life. What were you doing? If you were with others, who were they? What factors contributed to your happiness?

(b) Think of a time, you were proud. Why were you proud? Did others share your pride, who? What factors contributed to your pride?

(c) When have you been fulfilled and satisfied? What desire was fulfilled? How did the experience give your life meaning? What other factors contributed to your feelings of satisfaction?

Step 2:

(d) Based on these questions, list your values. Then prioritize them.

Step 3:

(e) Reaffirm your values by asking: do these values make you feel good about yourself? Are you proud of the top three you have chosen? Would you be comfortable and proud to tell those you respect and admire? Do these values represent you, even if it is not the most common values for others?

1.3 Beliefs

Beliefs are different from values (□ Table 1.1). Beliefs are the essence of how people see themselves, others, the world, and the future (Merriam-Webster's 1999). Core beliefs can both positively and negatively impact one's interpretation of social interaction. Taking the time to consider which beliefs are essential to you is a critical step in self-assessment. Once you understand your beliefs, you can identify:

━ What must you have in your career to grow and develop?

━ What would you like to have in your career, but isn't necessary for your career to grow and develop?

━ What is least important to you?

1.4 Skills

》 If you do not have the time to do it right, when will you find the time to do it over?

Skills are defined as the expertise needed to do a job (Merriam-Webster's 1999). Different types of skills exist, which can be divided into two categories: hard and soft.

◘ **Table 1.1** Values and beliefs comparison

Values	Beliefs
Principles or standards of behavior	Conviction or acceptance that something exists or is
The judgment of what is essential in	true, often without evidence
life	Affects your morals and values
Affects behavior and character	Some examples: "God created the world," "cheating is
Some examples: courage, respect,	immoral," or "lying is bad."
compassion	Often relates to religious or spiritual beliefs
Relates to everyday life	

Mckay (2019)

1.4.1 Hard Skills

Hard skills are easily measured. They consist of facts learned during formal education or training. Hard skills include technical expertise such as the ability to care for a patient on a ventilator or complete a patient medical history assessment.

1.4.2 Soft Skills

Soft skills are more challenging to measure. They are less tangible. A person acquires soft skills during life experiences. Examples of soft skills include communication abilities and interpersonal skills. The skills acquired during life experiences can lead to a career. For example, if a parent is a musician and teaches their child how to navigate in the music industry and how to sing. The acquired skills may lead to an eventual music career.

When considering what skills are needed in your identified nursing career path, you should explore what skills are required in order to be successful in that specific field of nursing. For example, if you are interested in becoming a hospice nurse, you may want to evaluate how you feel about working with not only patients but families. Hospice nurses work with patients at the end of life where significant others and families are typically intimately involved. Their work includes caring for dying patients and their families. If you are interested in this holistic approach to nursing and feel you have the soft skills for this nursing field, it may be an area you should consider.

In contrast to hospice nursing, if you are interested in becoming a certified registered nurse anesthetist (CRNA), you may want to evaluate how you feel about working in operating rooms where the patients are typically not awake. The environment is fast-paced, and the education required for this field of nursing requires training beyond a bachelor's degree in nursing (a doctoral degree in nursing is required). If you have the soft skills for working in a fast-paced, highly technical field of nursing, and the perseverance to complete many years of nursing education, CRNA may be an area you should consider.

Consider the following questions. Write your responses in a journal.

(a) What technical skills can you develop that would enhance your current position or help you expand your skillset for future career development? Some examples include improving your public speaking, writing, negotiation, or project planning skills.

(b) What competencies can you develop that would enhance your current position or help you expand your skills for future career development? Some examples include flexibility, time management, stress management, or assertiveness.

(c) What areas of self-management or personal growth would enhance your ability to develop your career path? Some examples include goal setting, decision-making, confidence in taking charge, or leadership skills.

1.5 Vision

Vision is a plan, mission, and direction for your life. It is your brand. It is your philosophy and what you feel you would like to become in life. This process is internal and comes from self-reflection and thought. The development of a vision requires understanding yourself first. You must know yourself and not try to copy others. You may want to adopt other people's vision but, ultimately, it should be your vision.

» Your vision drives your purpose.

The goal of developing a vision is to see your vision in detail and strive to achieve your vision. If you are not sure where to start, consider, are you drawn to technology and fascinated by the opportunities technologies bring us? Are you drawn to bringing order in chaotic situations or more regularity every day? Are you energized more by working with very young or very old? Once you successfully identify your vision, or your direction in life you are beginning to identify your brand.

There are several strategies one can use when developing a personal vision statement. Using your journal complete the following:

(a) Write down your vision statement. First, assess your needs, values, and interests. Provide yourself with adequate time to reflect and write down ideas as they come to you. Be sure to write nouns that describe you as a person (e.g., registered nurse (RN), parent, volunteer)

(b) Next, write down verbs associated with your vision (e.g. teach, runner, helps others, reader, writer).

(c) Next, visualize a picture of how you envision a perfect world. For example, "A perfect world is a place where no one suffers," or "everyone has enough money."

(d) Lastly, combine all the elements you reflected on and wrote above. An example of a vision, "my vision is to be an educator and to be known for inspiring students to be the best they can be."

1

Once you complete the evaluation of your values, beliefs, skills, and vision, you can begin to self-assess where you may want to go in your nursing career. Alignment of your career with your values, beliefs, skills, and vision can lead to satisfaction, fulfillment, and a sense of happiness. If you misalign your career with your values, beliefs, skills, and vision, you run the risk of minor to major problems. Problems could include misery, depression, or physical illness (Loffredo 2017). Identification and exploration of your values, beliefs, skills, and vision are part of a self-awareness journey. This journey should be intentional.

There are many resources available to assist in a self-awareness journey. Johnson and Johnson© (2019) has an online quiz to help a person evaluate where they want to go on their nursing career journey. The quiz begins with the following statements:

- I am thinking about nursing school
- I am in nursing school
- I am a nurse

As one works through the questions, they are assisted in directing you on your career journey and aligning a nursing specialty that fits with your interests. The resource can be found by going to the following link: ▶ https://nursing.jnj.com/find-my-specialty/

1.6 Personal Strengths and Weaknesses

》 I am only one: but still I AM ONE. I cannot do everything, but I can still do something. And because I cannot do everything, I will not refuse to do the something that I CAN DO. —Helen Keller

》 The biggest communication problem is we do not listen to understand. We listen to reply. —Bernard Shaw

Strengths are personal attributes cultivated over time. They may include a positive attitude, a willingness to learn, flexibility, integrity, dependability, friendliness, persistence, etc. Weaknesses are shortcoming, and knowing your weaknesses demonstrates how well you know yourself. When you know your weaknesses, you can take steps to improve. Weaknesses can include a skill which has not been learned, such as computer skills or training with a specialized piece of equipment. Another type of weakness could be poor communication or social skills. Specific examples could include poor organization, low patience, risk-taking, too much honesty, poor delegation, lack of creativity, and little flexibility. Weaknesses in interpersonal skills could consist of being too sensitive, too critical of others, frustration with under-performing colleagues, or confrontational.

One can make the most of talents through a personal SWOT analysis (Osterwalder and Pigneur 2010). SWOT refers to an analysis of strengths, weaknesses, analysis of opportunities, and threats that flow from them. SWOT is a useful tool that can assist in uncovering opportunities that would otherwise possibly remain hidden and prevent personal growth. A personal SWOT analysis can

Fig. 1.1 SWOT (Osterwalder and Pigneur 2010)

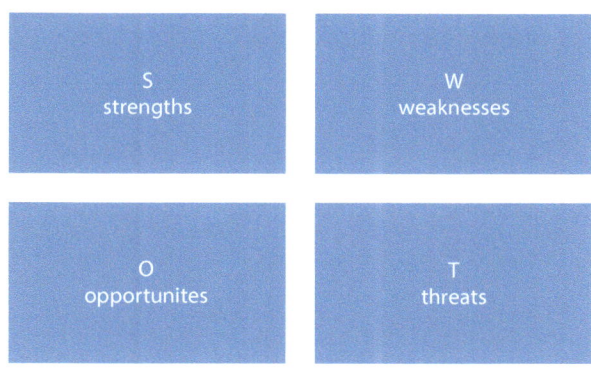

| S strengths | W weaknesses |
| O opportunites | T threats |

Consider the following questions as you evaluate your strengths. Write them in your journal.

• Do you have any advantages when you compare yourself to others? These may include education, skills, connections, etc.

• Do you "do" something well (when compared to others)?

• What do others see as your strengths? (You can ask them!)

• What values do you feel others fail to show?

• What achievements which make you proud?

• Do you have connections with others? Who are they? What is their expertise?

Fig. 1.2 SWOT—strengths analysis (Osterwalder and Pigneur 2010)

quickly be conducted by examining the following questions in an objective way and from your perspective (■ Fig. 1.1).

Strength is where you excel. It is your unique qualities that set you apart from others. For example, do people describe you as a caring person? Do they describe you as well-organized? Are you known for being adaptable or flexible? These strengths separate you from others and are part of your unique brand (■ Figs. 1.2 and 1.3).

Weaknesses are areas where can improve. For example, do you know that you become easily stressed in highly uncertain times, or do you adjust? Are you a very social person, or do you prefer to work alone? Do you fear talking in front of large groups of people? Do you dislike formal education training programs? Knowing your weaknesses helps you understand what drives you. While you can work on your weaknesses and improve them, this work will require motivation and perseverance (■ Figs. 1.4 and 1.5).

Opportunities are external factors that can give you an advantage. For example, do you know people who work in the field where you want to build your career eventually? Do you have a reliable support system to help you while you are in school or studying for a certification? These opportunities can help give you an advantage, which results in the increased likelihood of being successful on your journey (■ Fig. 1.6).

1

Interpersonal	Work ethic	Soft skills	Hard skills	Academics
• Compassion • Optimism • Delegates • Fair • Patience • Courage • Critical thinking • Communicates • Accepts constructive criticism	• Loyal • On time • Committed • Reliable • Able to handle multiple projects at one time • Recognizes others • Doesn't overextend oneself • Knows when good enough • Work/life balance	• Creative • Delegates • Organized • Impartial	• Computer literate • Bilingual • Competency	• Strong grammar and writing skills • Focused • Good test-taking skills • Good study skills

☐ **Fig. 1.3**   Examples of strengths (Osterwalder and Pigneur 2010)

Consider the following questions as you evaluate your personal weaknesses:

• What do you avoid because you feel a lack of confidence?

• What do others see as your weaknesses?

• What area of your skills/education do you feel are your weakest?

• Do you have negative work habits? What are they? (ex. poor stress management, persistently late, disorganization)

• Do you have personality weaknesses? Ex. Fear of public speaking, fear of leading, fear of conflict?

• You can ask others for input here. Observe how you compare to others' performance.

☐ **Fig. 1.4**   SWOT—weaknesses analysis (Osterwalder and Pigneur 2010)

Interpersonal	Work ethic	Soft skills	Hard skills	Academics
• Confrontational • Covers for others • Expects too much from others • Frustration with underperformance of others • Fear of public speaking • Critical of others • Internalizes others problems • Overly sensitive	• Does not finish projects • Too detailed • Too much multitasking • Take credit for group work • Take on too much at once • Too detail oriented • Perfectionist • Procrastinator • Works too much	• Not creative • Poor delegation • Poor organization • Impatient • Risk taker • Overly honest	• Poor Computer literacy • Doesn't speak foreign language • Poor speller • Poor writer • Lack technical knowledge in an area of patient care	• Challenged in a course • Poor writing skills • Overly involved in activities • Spends too much time on assignments • Challenged with standardized tests

Fig. 1.5 Examples of weaknesses (Osterwalder and Pigneur 2010)

Consider the following questions as you evaluate your opportunities?

• Is there something you need to understand better? Ex. Technology, networking, policy?

• Where is your current industry going? Are you taking advantage of the current market and future trends?

• Do you have a network of mentors who can advise you?

• How does your organization compare to competitors? Are there areas of weakness?

• Is there a need in your organization that no one is filling?

• Are their consistent complaints from customers in your company? Do you have a solution?

• Some strategies to address opportunities include learning new information through networking, education, or professional development. Do you need to advance a skill? Such as speaking, conflict management. When you look at your strengths, weaknesses, or opportunities, do you see any opportunities which open up if gaps were addressed?

Fig. 1.6 SWOT—opportunities analysis (Osterwalder and Pigneur 2010)

1

Consider the following as you evaluate your threats:

• Do you face any significant work obstacles?

• Are you in competition at your work for a project or a new role?

• Is your job changing?

• Is technology threatening your job?

• Are your weaknesses a threat? If so, which ones?

• By answering these questions, you can identify what you need to work on and put problems in the forefront of your perspective and assist with focus on improving you.

◻ **Fig. 1.7**   SWOT—threats analysis (Osterwalder and Pigneur 2010)

Threats are factors that can result in harm. For example, do you have numerous responsibilities in your personal life, which may take up your time when pursuing a new career? Do you have weaknesses you may not be able to overcome, such as a disability? Do you live far from a college or hospital where you want to work? Threats can be addressed and overcome. They are barriers we face, not deal-breakers. Understanding your threats helps you decide on the best career path, which is most likely to lead to success (◻ Fig. 1.7).

A SWOT analysis is a great way to guide personal career development. It requires the identification of strengths and weaknesses. It then moved to the identification of opportunities and threats. Following this analysis, one can brainstorm ideas and envision using the information you may not have been previously aware of before this personal SWOT exploration. Through SWOT analysis, one can develop a strategy for career development and filter down what needs to be done to be successful (Osterwalder and Pigneur 2010).

1.7 Self-Awareness

Self-awareness was first theorized in 1972 by Duval and Wicklund in the book, *A Theory of Objective Self Awareness*. The book explores the vital need to focus our attention on ourselves in an "inward" fashion. Self-awareness is a personal development tool and facilitates an understanding of values, strengths, weaknesses, habits, and why we react in a certain way. Those with strong self-awareness are best able to guide their future by controlling their reactions and behaviors through awareness. They can focus on their emotions and reactions. They are more "in control."

There are two types of self-awareness: internal and external. Internal self-awareness is how we see our values, reaction, fit with our environment, and our impact on others. Those with high levels of internal self-awareness are more likely to be successful in their jobs and relationships. External self-awareness is how others view our values, reactions, fit with the environment, and our impact. Those with high levels of external self-awareness have more empathy and more willing to

☐ **Fig. 1.8** Types of self-awareness (Eurich 2018)

Internal self awareness	External self awareness
• Clarity regarding "who you are" • Know what you want to accomplish	• Focus on appearing a certain way to others • Value others opinions

understand others' perspectives. Employees are often more satisfied with those with high levels of external self-awareness. Many people believe their self-awareness is strong; unfortunately, they overestimate this ability. The ☐ Fig. 1.8 above maps the two self-awareness types.

Self-awareness is a necessary process to help us understand ourselves. Knowing yourself helps you to understand how external factors affect you. You can then use this knowledge to be your best self and develop. A strong sense of self-awareness can guide the journey on your career path. Self-awareness will guide where you need to build your skills, self-discovery, and uncover bias. Self-awareness can improve your skills as a registered nurse (RN) by enhancing your ability to create a therapeutic environment for patients and in your communication with others. The power of becoming more self-aware is a journey, and you must travel down the path of personal self-improvement if you aim to improve your self-awareness.

Case Example 1.4 Self-Awareness Strategies

To become more self-aware, you must consistently do the following.
- Look at yourself objectively
- Keep a journal
- Write goals, plans, and prioritize
- Self-reflect every day
- Mediate and perform mindfulness techniques
- Complete personality tests
- Ask trusted friends and colleagues to describe you (Eurich 2018)

Once you build your self-awareness, you will find you are more confident and creative. You will make better decisions, build stronger relationships, and communicate more effectively.

1.8 Emotional Intelligence (EI)

Most of us recall a specific emphasis on evaluating our intelligence during our time in school when we took courses like Math and English. Historically, intelligence

◨ **Fig. 1.9**   Goleman emotional intelligence characteristics (Goleman 1995)

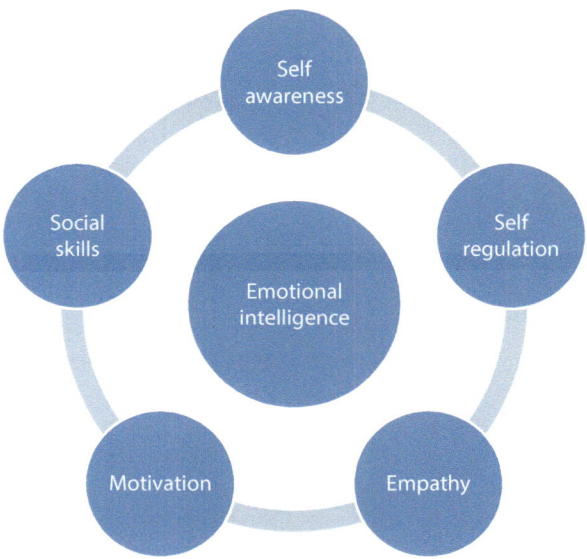

quotient (IQ) was the best way to measure academic performance and, ultimately, personal and professional success. For some time, research has been conducted to validate this belief. Recent findings have revealed that IQ plays a role but doesn't explain the reasons for personal success. IQ accounts for 25% of success in one's career. Emotional intelligence (EI) is another element in career success, which may be more important than IQ.

Daniel Goleman popularized emotional intelligence (EI) in his publication, *Emotional Intelligence*, published in 1995, based on years of research. Mr. Goleman aimed to investigate why some people were more successful than others in work and life and why they were successful. He concluded that Emotional Intelligence (EI) consists of five essential characteristics. They include self-awareness, self-regulation, empathy, motivation, and social skills (◨ Fig. 1.9).

By definition, Emotional Intelligence (EI) is the ability to manage one's emotions as well as other's emotions, especially in sensitive situations. An emotionally intelligent person has the ability to:

— Manage other people's emotions
— Regulate their own emotions
— Understand how their emotions impact others
— Know how to interpret their emotions
— Identify what they are feeling (Goleman 1995)

Emotional Intelligence (EI) can be naturally inherited, but it can also be developed through practice. The practice includes adapting the Emotional Intelligence (EI) characteristics to ensure they help promote emotional intelligence.

■ **Emotional Intelligence (EI) Characteristic: Self-Awareness**

Self-awareness includes self-confidence. Self-awareness was the title of this chapter and has been described in depth. From an emotional intelligence perspective, self-

■ **Fig. 1.10** Self-awareness (Goleman 1995)

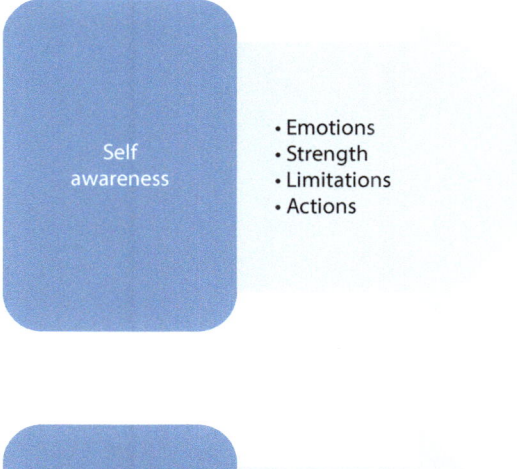

■ **Fig. 1.11** Self-management (Goleman 1995)

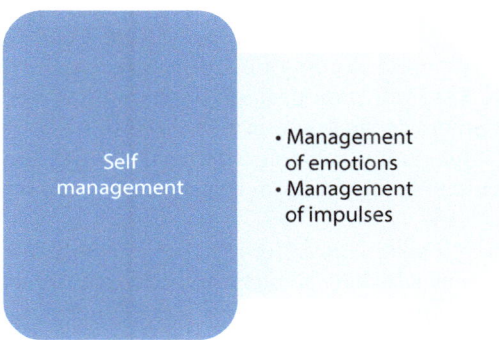

awareness is the ability to recognize four concepts: your emotions, strengths, limitation, and actions. One must understand how these concepts affect others around you. The benefit of self-awareness is you not only handle constructive criticism well, but you use it constructively to improve yourself. You begin to know your strengths and weaknesses and use this knowledge to improve yourself and your job performance. For example, in my job, I travel a lot, and my major weakness is a "poor sense of direction." Armed with this understanding, I overplan when I need to know where I am going. I invest more time planning how I will get where I need to go, and I allow much more time than is necessary to get there (■ Fig. 1.10).

■ **Emotional Intelligence (EI) Characteristic: Self-Management**

Self-management includes self-control. Self-management is the ability to manage your emotions and impulses wisely. Through self-management, you show restraint or show helpful emotions in certain situations. For example, when you are stressed, through self-regulation, you can better express yourself or recognize you need a break to recompose yourself. The benefit of self-management is that you earn trust and respect from others. You can use self-management when adapting to change. Self-management helps you to react rationally in stressful situations. Self-management can be improved by taking responsibility when a mistake is made. Do not blame others. When you admit your mistakes, you feel less guilty, and others form respect about you (■ Fig. 1.11).

1

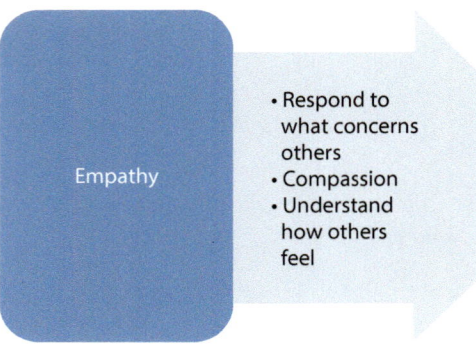

- **Emotional Intelligence (EI) Characteristic: Empathy**

Empathy is the ability to identify and understand others' emotions. It is the ability to imagine yourself in another's position. The benefits of empathy are the development of understanding how others feel and explain why they behave the way they do. Through empathy, you build compassion for others. You are more likely to help others because you genuinely respond to what concerns them. Empathy is helpful when delivering constructive feedback. Empathy shows caring. When you show empathy, you become respected, and your job performance improves (◻ Fig. 1.12).

To develop your empathy, imagine a person and their position. Even if you have not experienced what they have experienced, remember a situation where you felt like the way they feel, and identify the emotion you felt. The following strategies can be used to develop empathy:

— Practice active listening without interruption.
— Observe others and try to understand how they feel.
— Do not ignore other emotions. If someone looks upset, you need to acknowledge it and address it.
— Try first to understand, not judge. You may feel your own emotions build-up but instead, try to understand, you will be more empathic.
— Communicate with others using body language to regulate your body positions and your voice to demonstrate sincerity and an open listening style (Cherrry 2019).

- **Emotional Intelligence (EI) Characteristic: Social Skills**

People with social skills are easy to talk to. They are good listeners, patient, consistent, and predictable. Effective social skills are a way of managing relationships. The benefit of practical social skills is to build rapport with others and earn their respect. Respect and trust from others are key when unpopular decisions are made, as respect and trust will be needed. When your interest aligns with others, identify their individual needs, and determine how their abilities can be used to best. Make others comfortable in discussing their concerns (◻ Fig. 1.13).

Fig. 1.13 Social skills
(Goleman 1995)

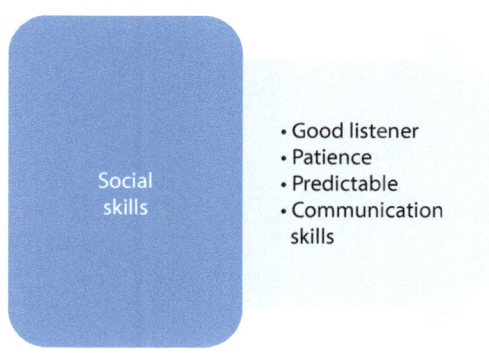

Social
skills

• Good listener
• Patience
• Predictable
• Communication
  skills

One can build effective social skills by:

— Improving communication skills such as ensuring clarity, conciseness, coherence, correctness, careful consideration and confidence (**Fig. 1.14**). When there are problems, poor communication and misunderstandings upset others. Listen to feedback from others and work out a manager to speak with the intent of open body language and active listening.
— Learn to provide praise and constructive feedback.
— Work cooperatively towards a shared goal.
— Listen and practice empathy.
— Build relationships and assist in understanding each person based on their individuality.
— Resolve conflict by looking at the situation from all viewpoints and work towards a compromise (**Fig. 1.13**).

■ **Emotional Intelligence (EI) Characteristic: Motivation**

Motivation is moving towards the achievement of goals. This moving towards goals includes drive, commitment to a group or organization's goals, initiative, and optimism despite obstacles. Motivation first comprises the *activation* of a goal or the decision to do something. Next, motivation includes *intensity* or the amount of effort that is going into doing something. Lastly, *perseverance* is the amount of time you can keep up your motivational efforts (**Fig. 1.15**). Achieving a goal requires all of the above components. Some people are good at activating but not perseverance. Recognition of this variation in motivational skills is critical in determining success in reaching goals.

The benefits of motivation are:

— Less procrastination
— More self-confidence
— More motivation, even in the face of challenges
— Focus on goal achievement

The above behaviors are contagious to others, and they will adopt them. Motivational behaviors influence others to do the same. To develop your self-motivation, consider why you do the job you do. Think about the way you sought

1

■ **Fig. 1.14** The 6 C's of communication (▶ http://www.fsb.miamioh.edu/fsb/content/programs/howe-writing-initiative/HWI-handout-CsofBusComm.html)

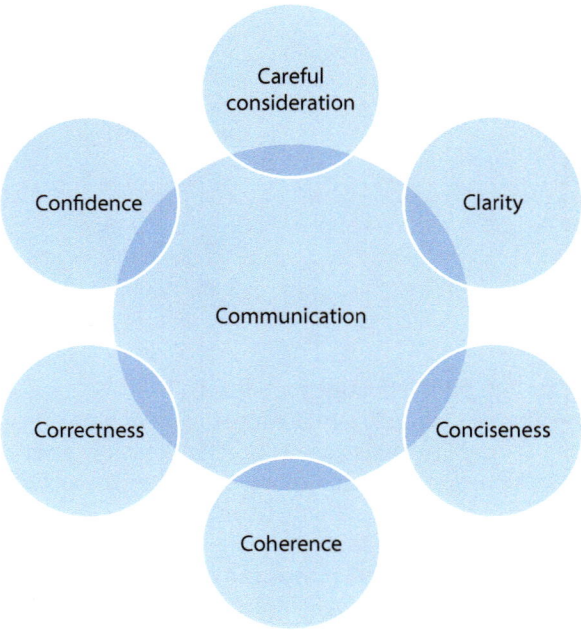

■ **Fig. 1.15** What is motivation? (Goleman 1995)

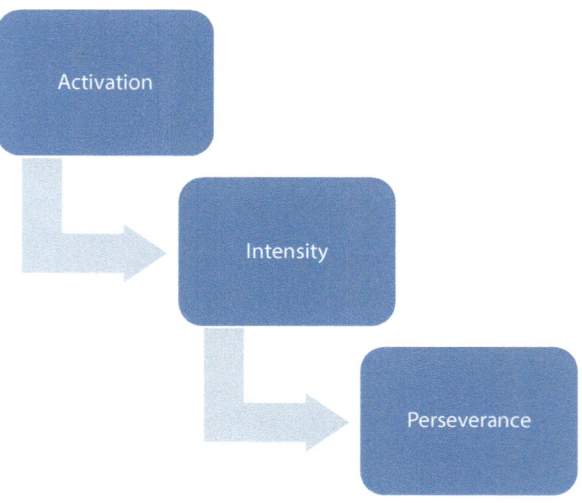

it initially. Set goals. Consistently act on them and revise as needed. Be optimistic and decisive, even in the face of challenges. Tell others why your goals are valuable to you, which provides you with an ongoing sense of purpose.

Emotional Intelligence (EI) can be developed. Many books are available to help you explore Emotional Intelligence (EI) concepts, assess yourself, and identify your strengths and weaknesses.

1.9 Conclusion

The self-assessment chapter explored many concepts about oneself. It is essential to understand that while this book explores the process of building a successful nursing career, building your successful career requires first, looking inward, as this process is unique, your own.

Through this process of plotting your career path and following inward reflection, the road to building a *meaningful,* successful nursing career is beginning. One may notice, there has been little to no mention of nursing careers thus far, this is intentional as self-awareness may lead you down a different path.

■ **Activities**
Complete these free online quizzes:

? Activity 1
Emotional Intelligence Test by Psychology Today. This test takes 45 minutes. You can receive a free summary report. Am I emotionally intelligent? ► https://www.psychologytoday.com/us/tests/personality/emotional-intelligence-test

? Activity 2
PositivePsychology.com offers 17 emotional intelligence tests and assessments you can complete for free. ► https://positivepsychology.com/emotional-intelligence-tests/

Strategies
There are many strategies and free tools online to assist with developing some of the concepts introduced in this chapter. Below are some strategies:
1. Consider—what is most important to you. Do your choices about how, where, and with whom you spend your time reflect what is important to you?
2. Self-awareness quiz: The internet offers many short quizzes to help define certain concepts. Questionnaires to assess self-awareness are no different, and there are many online quizzes out there.
3. ProProfs.com is an internet site with software tools. The site includes a free online self-awareness quiz, which aims to give the participant an idea of how self-aware they are. The questionnaire takes a couple of minutes and consists of 10 questions. Upon completion, you obtain an assessment of your self-awareness with a brief evaluation and tips for improving your self-awareness.

ProProfs Quizzes. Quiz: How self-aware are you? ► https://www.proprofs.com/quiz-school/story.php?title=how-selfaware-are-you, there are ten questions. This quiz will give you an idea of how self-aware you are.
4. Self-awareness improvement strategies
   ‒ Keep a reflection diary. Write down situations you have experienced and focus on the emotions you expressed. Express your thoughts and behaviors during the circumstances. Use this information to understand your emotions and reactions. Work towards improved self-regulation.

1

- Ask for feedback from people you trust. Use their feedback to help you improve your reactions in the future.
- Observe the responses of others. Begin to evaluate their behaviors and identify their strengths and weaknesses in their self-awareness.

5. An emotional intelligence test. This online test is offered by Psychology Today and takes 45 minutes to complete. You receive a free summary evaluation and can pay to have a more in-depth set of results, but this is not necessary. You must be honest when completing this quiz to ensure the results are as accurate as possible.

Psychology Today Emotional Intelligence Test: ▶ https://www.psychologytoday.com/us/tests/personality/emotional-intelligence-test

6. Improve body language. There are online body language tests to help you evaluate interactions with others. Body language often says more than the spoken word. This quiz will help indicate your understanding of body language. Psychtests: Body Language Test: ▶ https://testyourself.psychtests.com/testid/3764 You will receive an interpretation of your score.

Vignettes
Vignette 1
I like nursing because it's a profession that never stops giving. You learn new things every day, and the opportunity for growth is almost unlimited. I feel so good inside when I see improvement in my patients and also when giving emotional support by holding the hands of family members who have just experienced tragedy. It gives me an inner peace that I was able to help somebody.

My mom told me every time you have patients and family members, and they feel better, count that as a blessing. I'm still counting my blessings every day, and–guess what?—I'm getting paid for that. I thank God every day for this opportunity I have been given.

Vignette 2
What are your strengths in nursing?
My strongest skill is patient education. It can soften fears and improve outcomes. One patient was unable to reduce his blood pressure following a heart attack. I was tasked with helping educate him about diet and exercise. I sourced some video case studies about patients just like him who'd changed their routines. Three months later he wrote me a letter. His blood pressure and lipid profile were all down into a healthy range.

References

Cherry (2019) Understanding body language and facial expressions. Very well mind. Retrieved from: https://www.verywellmind.com/understand-body-language-and-facial-expressions-4147228

Eurich T (2018) What self awareness really is (and how to cultivate it) Harvard Business Review. Retrieved from: https://hbr.org/2018/01/what-self-awareness-really-is-and-how-to-cultivate-it

Goleman D (1995) Emotional intelligence. Bantam Dell, New York

List of weaknesses with examples. The balance careers. https://www.thebalancecareers.com/list-of-weaknesses-2063805

Loffredo S (2017) Do your career and work values align? Inside Higher Education. Retrieved from: https://www.insidehighered.com/advice/2017/11/13/importance-aligning-your-career-your-core-values-essay

Mckay (2019) Self assessment. The balance careers. https://www.thebalancecareers.com/self-assessment-524753

Merriam-Webster's (1999) Merriam-Webster's collegiate dictionary, 10th edn. Merriam-Webster Incorporated, Springfield

Osterwalder A, Pigneur Y (2010) Business model generation: a handbook for visionaries, game changes, and challenges. Wiley.

Self Assessment by McGill Career Planning Service. https://www.mcgill.ca/caps/students/explore/self-assessment

Self-assessment skills. UC Berkeley. https://hr.berkeley.edu/development/career-development/self-assessment/skills

What are your values? Deciding what's most important in life. Mind Tools. https://www.mindtools.com/pages/article/newTED_85.htm

What is self-awareness and how to develop it? Devel Good habits: a better life one habit at a time. https://www.developgoodhabits.com/what-is-self-awareness/

Goal Setting and Self-Discipline

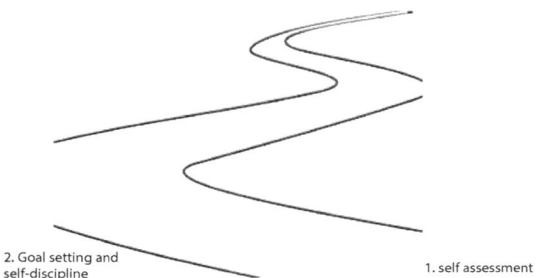

2. Goal setting and self-discipline

1. self assessment

Contents

© Springer Nature Switzerland AG 2020
J. M. Manning, *The Path to Building a Successful Nursing Career*,
https://doi.org/10.1007/978-3-030-50023-8_2

All who have accomplished great things have had a high aim, have fixed their gaze on a high goal, one which sometimes seemed impossible. —Orison Swett Marden

Regarding self-discipline: "you can never conquer the mountain; you can only conquer yourself" —Jum Whittaker

» It's never too late to be what you might have been. —George Eliot, English Novelist

2.1 Goal Setting

» A goal without a plan is just a wish —Antoine de Saint-Exupery

Many people feel adrift in the world. They work hard but don't seem to get anywhere worthwhile. Is this you? Do you ask why do others achieve so much more than me? Did you know that one reason you feel this way is that you haven't spent enough time thinking about what you want from your life? You haven't set formal goals. Ask yourself, would you set out on a long journey with no idea of your destination and how you would get there? Goal setting used by successful professionals such as top-level athletes, successful business people, high achievers in all fields. The goals must be clearly defined. Goal setting includes taking steps to develop oneself.

Ongoing progress evaluation is necessary when setting goals. You must motivate yourself towards the achievement of goals. These concepts are fundamental in the achievement of goals that are long term. When you set goals, you improve self-confidence.

Consider a goal you wanted to achieve in the past. Maybe you tried to lose weight, consider this example. Consider the challenges in reaching this goal. Did you want to lose 10 or 100 lbs? You could not achieve this goal by wishing it to happen; you had to work for it. Setting the goal may have been difficult. How quickly do I want to lose weight? What is realistic? Once the goal was set, a plan was needed, and ongoing motivation was required. Will I join a program like weight watchers, or will I do this myself? Little setbacks may have occurred, but they did not prevent you from reaching a final goal. You may have diverted from your purpose during the holidays or your vacation, but you got back on track afterward.

Goal setting is a powerful process and gets you to think about the future. It can motivate you and turn a vision into reality. Setting goals helps you choose where you want to go in life. You set exact goals which align with what you want to achieve and where to concentrate your efforts. Through goal setting, distractions can be identified quickly to ensure you are not led astray.

2.2 Lifetime Goal Setting: Where Do You Want to Be in the Future?

2

>> Start with the end in mind —Franklin Covey

Lifetime goal setting is an excellent place to start. You must first consider what you want to achieve in your lifetime or by some distant age in the future. Life goals are more than "what you want to achieve to survive." Carefully constructed life goals can guide daily goals, short-term goals, and long-term behaviors. A lifetime goal is personal ambition and provides a sense of direction in life.

Why set goals? Goals clarify behaviors; they put our attention on something to focus our efforts. Goals allow us to assess where we are, where we want to be, and the progress in getting there. Goals can provide meaning and purpose. Goals allow us to focus on our strengths, resulting in an increase in confidence and increased likelihood of achieving goals. One place to start is to reflect on areas beyond your career. Consider areas such as family, education, finances, career, attitude, physical, service, and hobbies. ◘ Table 2.1 describes some questions you can use to guide this reflection in determining your lifetime goals.

These visionary questions are intended to help you brainstorm and reflect on your goals. You should take the time to explore then identify a couple of goals to focus on specifically. Practical goals must be unique to you and based on your values and beliefs (► Chap. 1). They should not reflect what others want for you. There are many choices when considering lifetime goals. One must remember the path must be sought out; it will not appear before you. The door you want to open must be intentionally pursued, it will not appear before you and beg you to open it.

Take the time to talk with those working in areas you are interested in, ask them questions about their work, benefits, pros and cons, and typical work week. Know your interests—social or work with small groups. What patient populations do you enjoy the most? Do you enjoy a fast pace or working overtime in a challenging environment?

Case Example: Allison

Let's consider the same case example through the next sections of ► Chap. 2. Allison wants to become a Board-Certified Pediatric Nurse Practitioner and open a nurse-run clinic. Betty is 25 years old and has been working as a waitress since high school. She received a general studies degree at her local university after high school and received pretty good grades. She did not know what to do with her degree, so she kept working as a waitress. Betty has set a lifetime goal, which will take her more than 5 years to accomplish. Tips on Choosing the Right Nursing Job (n.d.).

2.3 · Short-Term Goals: Where Do You Want to Be in the Next 5 Years?

27

2

□ Table 2.1 Considerations in forming lifetime goals (Patel 2020)

Using your journal create a subheading page for each of the major areas below. Reflect and document answers to the questions for each area

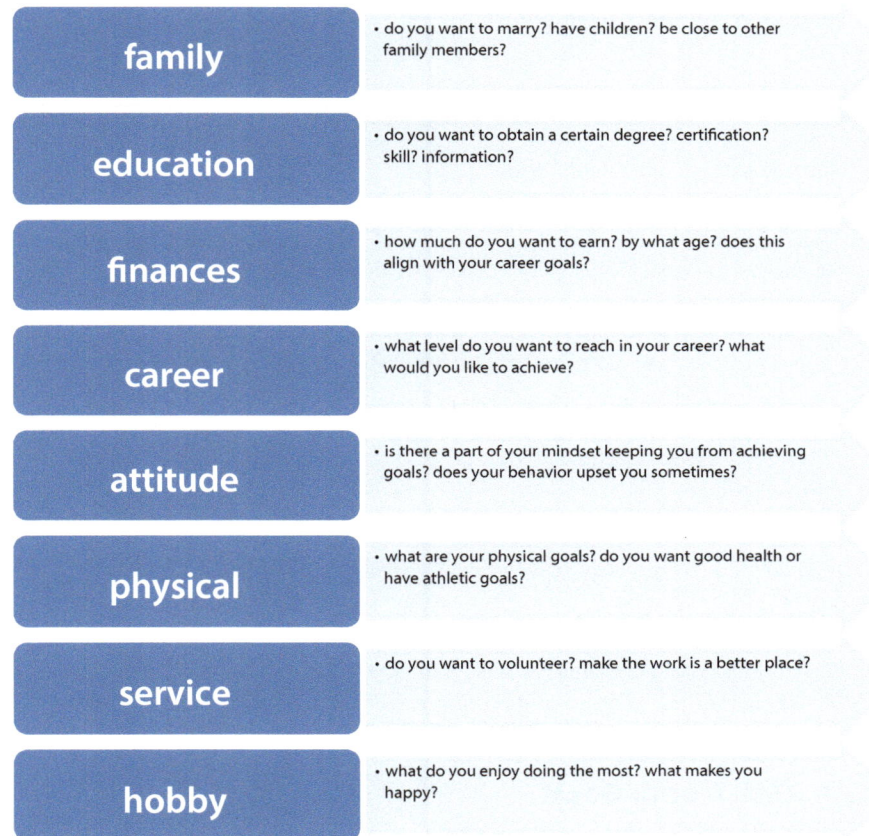

family	• do you want to marry? have children? be close to other family members?
education	• do you want to obtain a certain degree? certification? skill? information?
finances	• how much do you want to earn? by what age? does this align with your career goals?
career	• what level do you want to reach in your career? what would you like to achieve?
attitude	• is there a part of your mindset keeping you from achieving goals? does your behavior upset you sometimes?
physical	• what are your physical goals? do you want good health or have athletic goals?
service	• do you want to volunteer? make the work is a better place?
hobby	• what do you enjoy doing the most? what makes you happy?

2.3 Short-Term Goals: Where Do You Want to Be in the Next 5 Years?

Once you identify and describe your lifetime goals, you should identify and define your short-term goals (such as those achievable in 5 years or less). Next, 1 year, 6 months and a 1-month plan should be laid out in detail. Each goal

2

should align with each other and build upon each other. Now that you have listed your goals, you can create a "to-do" list. A "to-do" list could include obtaining more information through web searching, book reading, ted talks, etc. Through this list, you can begin setting out to achieve your successful career goals. Case Example 2.1 continues with the case example in describing the development of short term goals.

Case Example 2.1 Unfolding Case Example: Allison

Case Example Continued: Allison

Allison needs to set some 5-year goals. She decides she must become a Pediatric Nurse Practitioner (PNP) and establish herself before opening her clinic. She sets off to achieve this goal. Some goals for her 5-year plan include:

Year 1
1. Identify an RN school she wants to apply to (there are accelerated programs she can complete in 2 years and obtain her BSN)
2. Identify the requirements needed to apply to the program
3. Complete any necessary prerequisites requirements for the program
4. Apply for the RN program

Years 2–4
5. Attend the BSN program and obtain a degree in nursing
6. Identify prerequisites required for PNP program (typically 1-year RN experience with pediatric patients)

Years 4–5
7. Work in pediatric settings as an RN for 1 year
8. Apply for PNP program and begin studies

2.3.1 One-Month Goals

There are lots of 1-month goals for people to explore. Monthly goals can lead to significant life changes. The key is daily progress. Tim Robbins, a motivational speaker, cites that all results come from rituals. Case Example 2.2. continues with the case example in describing the development of monthly and 1 year goals.

Case Example 2.2 Unfolding Case Example: Allison

Case example continued: Allison

If you consider the case example, the first step for Allison is to explore which RN program she wants to attend and determine which prerequisites are needed to apply to the program. These goals can be completed in 1 month

Month 1

1. Conduct an online search of the accelerated RN programs in your area (evaluate 1–3 programs)
2. Identify which program to apply to in 2 weeks
3. Determine which prerequisites are needed for the identified RN program in 3 weeks
4. By the end of the month, decide what courses you need to take at what university before applying to the RN program selected

2.3.2 Six-Month Goals

Case Example Continued: Allison

In the case example, Allison needs to take several prerequisite courses before applying to the RN program; this goal can be put into action in 6 months where she can

1. Register for her prerequisite courses
2. Begin taking the courses
3. Complete the semester
4. Apply to RN program

Some things may not be in her control. For example, maybe the classes are not offered in the next available semester, or perhaps she needs to save money to pay for the courses. These challenges should not stop you from achieving your goal. Ensure your goals are written based on what you can control. For example, in goal two above, state, "begin taking courses in the first available semester"

2.3.3 One-Year Goals

Case Example Continued: Allison

Year-long goals may seem long term. They are not; they are goals that should connect to actual long-term goals (5-year goals and lifetime goals)

In the case example for Allison, her 1-year goals include

1. Apply to RN program
2. Increase hours at a job and save money for tuition and fees
3. Begin RN program

These goals can be completed in 1 year

2

■ **Fig. 2.1** Short-term goal setting (Patel 2020)

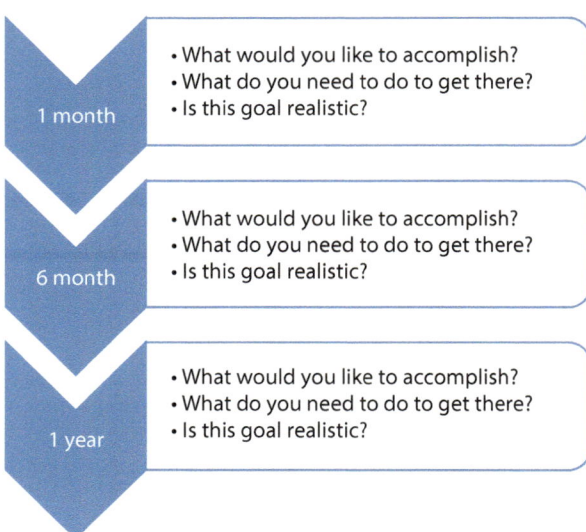

1 month
- What would you like to accomplish?
- What do you need to do to get there?
- Is this goal realistic?

6 month
- What would you like to accomplish?
- What do you need to do to get there?
- Is this goal realistic?

1 year
- What would you like to accomplish?
- What do you need to do to get there?
- Is this goal realistic?

When setting short-term goals, there are many considerations one needs to evaluate to ensure they are achievable. For example, one must ask what they would like to accomplish? What steps are required to reach the goal, and is the goal realistic? Is the time frame realistic? (■ Fig. 2.1).

It is important to frequently revisit your identified goals to ensure you are remaining on track. If you are not staying on track, revise as needed. You may need to put a reminder on your calendar to ensure you do this step. The path towards goal achievement is never perfect. You cannot predict or anticipate every step. The goals must be modified over time and adjusted. There will be unexpected obstacles, and sometimes things will move faster than expected. Some goals take longer than expected, some shorter. For example, if one of your goals is to choose a new hospital. Be sure to visit the hospital, look around, visit the nursing unit, observe the environment, observe the staff nurses, the patients, and the families. Consider asking for a tour by the recruiter. Talk with the staff at all levels. Talk to the staff at the bedside and administration. Are people smiling? Are they happy? Do things appear to be running smoothly?

2.3.3.1 **Where Are You Now?**

Now that goals are written down and described for the near and distant future, you should assess where you are now. In this process, you must recognize your interests and skills. You are tying interests and abilities to your goal-related concepts described in ▶ Chap. 1. For example, when you completed your self-assessment, you matched your preferences and explored options which were a good fit for you. You should assess aspects of your life, such as personal and work. Would you like to see a significant change for yourself in these areas?

2.3.3.2 Setting the Path to Achieving Future Goals

Setting the path to achieving goals is a time consuming and thoughtful process. It is intentional and does not occur "by chance." You must allow yourself the opportunity to consider your current situation and short-term goals. Write your goals using SMART goal principles (Murphy 2010).

2.3.4 SMART Goals

What does SMART goal mean?

SMART is an acronym used when developing a goal. George Doran coined the term in 1981 in his Management Review publication. Robert Rubin went on to write an article in Society for Industrial and Organization Psychology. The acronym, SMART, can be used to ensure goals are written clearly and measurably. Each letter in the SMART goal acronym describes essential elements of SMART goals (◘ Fig. 2.2).

2.3.4.1 S = Specific

A specific goal must be simple, significant, and sensible. When writing goals, one can ask the following questions: (1) What do I want to accomplish? (2) Why is this goal important? (3) Who is involved? (4) Where is it located and (5) Which resources or limits are required? Imagine where you want to go in your career. For example, if you're going to become a registered nurse. A specific goal could be, "I want to gain the skills and experience necessary to become a registered nurse."

2.3.4.2 M = Measurable

A measurable goal must be motivating and meaningful. A measurable goal is essential in tracking progress and staying focused. It ensures you will be more likely to meet deadlines and become engaged in achieving your goal. A measurable goal should address questions, such as (1) How much? (2) How many? and (3) How will I know I have accomplished my goal? For example, imagine you want to become a certified registered nurse. You may have time-bound factors to consider. A measurable goal considers these factors and could include, "I want to become critical care certified registered nurse in 2 years." The goal should be written in a time-bound

◘ Fig. 2.2 Setting SMART goals (Patel 2020)

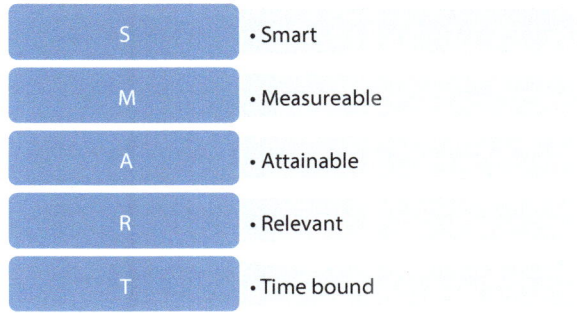

- S — • Smart
- M — • Measureable
- A — • Attainable
- R — • Relevant
- T — • Time bound

context that is realistic as it takes one 1 year of working experience to gain the hours needed to certify, and you have given yourself another year to study and take the certification exam.

2.3.4.3 A = Achievable

An achievable goal must be attainable. A goal needs to be realistic. It should stretch your current abilities but remain feasible. An achievable goal helps you identify opportunities or resources that can ensure your success in meeting the goal. An achievable goal should address questions such as (1) How can I accomplish this goal? and (2) How realistic is the goal for me? For example, if becoming a certified critical care registered nurse requires 1 year of critical care experience. Are you currently working in this type of field? If not, you may need to set your goal to include the time necessary to transition to this type of work environment. Another word of caution when setting a goal that you may not have control over, such as "I want to get promoted in 1 year," remember you may not be able to control this goal. A better goal maybe, "I want to obtain the experience and skills needed to be considered for a promotion in my current job."

2.3.4.4 R = Relevant

A relevant goal must be reasonable, realistic, and results-based. Your goals should matter to you and align with your lifetime and short-term goals. Support will be needed to achieve your goals. You must maintain control over them. Ensure your goal drives everyone forward. Relevant goals should address: (1) Does the goal seem worthwhile? (2) Is it the right time for this goal? (3) Does the goal match my other efforts and needs? (4) Am I the right person to reach this goal? and (5) Is my goal applicable in the current socio-economic environment? You may want to become a certified registered nurse and may find the time needed to transition to a critical care unit is not the right time right now. You may want to evaluate the organization's goals at this time. Maybe the organization is looking at expanding other departments. Perhaps you are considering starting a family, and transitioning to a new unit may complicate this goal. All these factors should be considered to ensure the goal is realistic and reasonable.

2.3.4.5 T = Time-Bound

A time-bound goal must be time-based, timely, time-sensitive, and time-limited. Recent literature has expanded SMART goals to describe SMARTER goals where the E = evaluated and R = reviewed. All purposes need a target deadline. This component is often missed in goal setting and results in goals that are not attained. This component of a SMART goal ensures you will remain focused and not become distracted by other everyday tasks you must achieve. Time-bound goals answer the following questions: (1) When (2) What can I do 6 months from now (3) what can I do 6 weeks from now and (4) what can I do today? In the case of becoming a certified registered nurse, one must consider how long it will take to complete the requirements realistically. Use those time frames to help in setting an appropriate time-bound goal.

SMART goals are useful in providing the motivation and focus needed to achieve goals. It helps improve the likelihood of goal achievement (❑ Fig. 2.2). A

SMART goal can help you find the real reason your goals have not been put into motion. They can help with creating a vision to achieve a long- or short-term goal. If you do not adhere to these elements, you risk setting goals that are not achievable and unlikely to be met.

Most goals fail due to poorly written goals and poor execution. The more active the goal, the more likely the chance of success in achieving the goal. Goal setting is a skill that can be learned. Ensure you set enough time to set goals and prioritize them to ensure they will be useful in your journey to building a successful nursing career.

2.3.5 Writing Your Goals

There are many tips for writing practical goals which lead to follow through and maximize chances for success. Consider lifetime goals you want to accomplish in life. Consider essential milestones needed to achieve this lifetime goal. Further, describe (actually write them down) these goals. State who will do these goals and when they will be done. Consider your goal fits in your lifetime goal. Ensure your goal aligns with your long-term strategies and connects to life goals. Ensure your goal is written with an action verb. State what you will do. Your goal should be understood by anyone who reads it. Also, realize you must own your goal, and you are ultimately accountable for the success of your goal. Ask yourself, if your goal defines success and prioritizes the goal. ◘ Table 2.2 describes some tips and rationales for the development of effective goals. These tips can serve as a checklist for the goals you have set to ensure you have set achievable goals. Good luck!

◘ **Table 2.2** Tips and rationales for development of effective goals (Patel 2020)

Tips	Rationale
Express goals positively	Stating what you don't want is not as effective
Be precise	Time, date, and amounts are essential components of an effective goal
Set priorities	Helps to focus attention and avoid feelings of being overwhelmed
Write them down	Visual reminders facilitate clarity and preciseness
Keep your goals visible	If you can see your goal, you can stay focused and accountable
Create long-term goals	A long-term goal is part of the larger plan, and your short-term plans should align with long-term goals
Break into small goals	Frequent successes promote motivation
Be realistic	Ensure a feeling of control over what you can achieve
Evaluate and revise	Evaluate the goals periodically and revise. It is ok to adjust goals when needed

2

2.4 Self-Discipline

» In reading about the lives of great people, I have found that the first victory won was over themselves —Harry Truman

Studies show those with self-discipline are happier. Why? They spend less time debating whether to do something and can make positive choices. The self-disciplined recognize impulses and feelings which direct their options and consider the pros and cons. Once making a disciplined decision, they have higher levels of satisfaction.

Self-discipline includes several strategies such as know your weaknesses, remove temptation, set clear goals with a path to achieve, take small steps, prioritize self discipline, do not accept excuses, avoid self entitlement and understand perfection may not be possible.

2.4.1 Know Your Weaknesses

Your weaknesses hold you back from achieving your goals. You have the power to improve your weaknesses, but only after you identify them. Learn from your failures. Don't fear failure. Many people fear failure so much they never try. The beautiful part about failure is that it shows you what you are doing wrong. You can learn what to do better and identify what changes are needed. A willingness to revise and change your goals based on realistic goal evaluation proves you are not willing to get up. Failure leads to new opportunities through experience. You learn more about yourself and how to modify and set better goals in the future for your self. Failure is a learning opportunity, not a setback in goal achievement.

2.4.2 Remove Temptation

The potential temptation must be recognized before it can be redirected and eliminated. You must be honest with your limitations and visualize yourself resisting temptation. Consider the long-term consequences and distract yourself from the temptation. Reduce the choice that you must make by removing the temptation. Don't procrastinate. Now is the moment. If you put off till later, you are giving up on doing what you want to do. Distractions are the enemy! Eliminate them. Find a comfortable space to focus and reflect. Surround yourself with like-minded individuals who can keep you grounded and focused. Don't let notifications on your phone distract you.

2.4.3 Set Clear Goals with a Path to Achieve

Goals must be clear and broken down into steps. Progress must be monitored and evaluated. Try to make the objective fun and celebrate your accomplishments along the way. In your goal setting, be careful not to expect things you cannot control. You cannot control how others will behave on your journey to success nor circumstances you could not anticipate. Be cautious of disappointment, frustration, or anger, as these will stop your motivation. Accept what you cannot always plan and redirect. Take a setback as a learning experience and improve the process. Remember to maintain as much consistency as possible. Work on your goal each day. Case Example 2.3 provides some examples of career goals.

Case Example 2.3 Example Career Goals: Family Nurse Practitioner

Goal: become a family nurse practitioner
 Objectives:
 1. Contact university for BSN and graduate program information and application materials
 2. Complete BSN program
 3. Obtain a job as an RN
 4. Schedule Graduate Record Examinations (GRE)
 5. Prepare for GRE
 6. Contact professionals for reference letters
 7. Complete forms and schedule physical exam
 8. Submit application materials on time
 9. Apply for financial aid (if applicable)
 10. Make an appointment with an academic advisor to plan course progression
 11. Register for courses

2.4.4 Take Small Steps

Create a plan and divide it into small steps. Taking small steps eliminates the fear of failure and procrastination. A big step is intimidating. Make your goals as small as you want, such as daily goals, hourly goals, weekly goals. Make a to-do list every day to help you stay accountable for your actions and help you focus on a visual target. A step in the right direction is a step towards your goal. Small rewards will go a long way in keeping you on your path.

2.4.5 Prioritize Self-Discipline

Set a schedule and stick to it. If you fall off your path, reflect, adjust, forgive yourself, and get back on track. Use tools to help you stay on your schedule. For example, calendars, smartphone apps, alarms, sticky notes, and to-do lists.

2.4.6 No Excuses

Stop the negative self-talk such as I am not ready, I am not good enough, It is not the right time, I do not have enough money, It is too hard, It will take too long, People will laugh at me, People will tell me I cannot do it. There are so many examples of negative self-talk. We are good at it. Your mind tends to keep you in a comfort zone, challenge this mindset, and venture into unchartered territory. Face the self-doubt. Practice self-affirmation every day. Look at yourself in the mirror and affirm your goals and your abilities. Use a journal to reinforce your thinking.

2

Silence negative thoughts and replace them with positive ones. Motivate yourself, only you can do it. Be fearless!

2.4.7 Avoid Self-Entitlement

Don't let your ego get in your way. It is easy to become self-entitled and believe you deserve success regardless of the work needed to achieve the goal. It is important to celebrate accomplishments along your path to success. Always remain grateful and humble during the process. There is still someone out there who is facing more challenges than you, and they remain thankful for what they have.

2.4.8 Perfection May Not Be Possible

You need to remember you cannot control everything. If you become frustrated with the journey, you can become disheartened. When the unexpected happens, take pause. Analyze the situation and ask yourself: Will this setback stop me from achieving the goal I have set? If the delay doesn't, adapt and move one. This process builds flexibility, adaptability, and creativity, as achieving goals is never seamless nor an entirely predictable path. ◘ Figure 2.3 describes some goal setting tips.

Create simple good habits
(a) Change your perception about your willpower
(b) Create a backup plan
(c) Reward yourself
(d) Forgive yourself and move forward
(e) Creating good habits
(f) Consistency

◘ **Fig. 2.3**   Goal-setting tips
(The University of California,
San Francisco 2020)

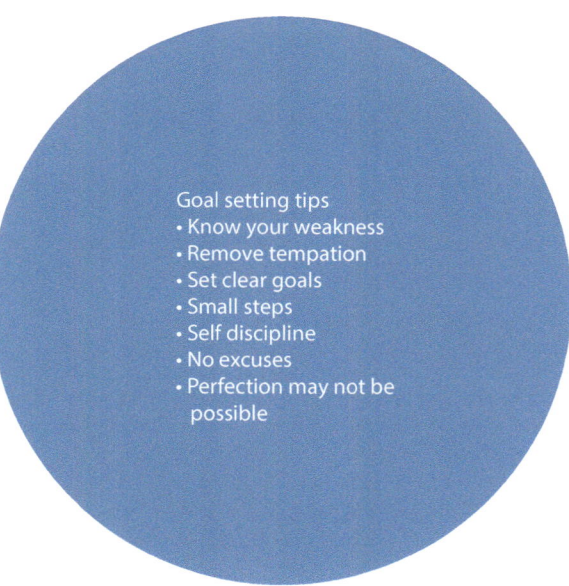

Goal setting tips
• Know your weakness
• Remove tempation
• Set clear goals
• Small steps
• Self discipline
• No excuses
• Perfection may not be
  possible

(g) Long-term vs. short-term thinking
(h) Organization
(i) Adaptability

■ **Activities**

Complete these free online quizzes:

? **Activity 1**

How good are your goals?
An online website, Mind Tools, offers a free quiz to explore one's goal-setting approach. Once completed, the participant receives a score and interpretation of goal setting. ► https://www.mindtools.com/pages/article/goal-setting-quiz.htm

? **Activity 2**

An online website, My personality, offers life goals test. This test provides users with insight into the realistic or unrealistic goals they have set. ► https://www.seemypersonality.com/personality.asp?p=Success-Test#q1

? **Activity 3**

Create a to-do list for today. Purchase a calendar and add activities for each day. Refer to your goals (both short term and long term). Ask yourself if your daily list and weekly activities align and bring you towards your short-term and long-term goals?

? **Activity 4**

Start a journal. Write down your core values. Write down your career goals. Do your values and goals align?

Strategies

Strategy 1. There are many strategies to ensure successful goal setting. The key is to identify which one works best for you.

1. Send a letter to future self on futureme.org. Users can send a message to their future self, which can be delivered in 1, 3, or year time frames. ► https://www.futureme.org/.
2. Write three goals you want to accomplish in the next 5 years and three goals you want to achieve in more than 5 years.
3. Write a list of your strengths and weaknesses. Write action items on how you can realistically overcome your weaknesses.

Strategy 2. Self-discipline can be mastered in many ways. Here are some tips for self-discipline.

1. Create an organizational system to manage time.
2. You can begin by writing down your weaknesses. Acknowledge them.
3. Establish a clear plan or strategy to eliminate bad habits.
4. Remove temptation. If you want to stop eating chips, stop buying chips.
5. Visualize long-term goals. See it, feel it.
6. Recover from mistakes with grace and effectiveness.

2

Vignettes
Vignette 1
Jim Carrey told a story once about his struggling days and how he daydreamed of success and imagined himself entertaining on a global level. In 1985, he wrote a check to himself for 10 million dollars for acting services rendered. The check dated for 10 years into the future. He kept the check. In 1995, he was offered 10 million dollars to make *Dumb and Dumber*. The take-home message here is if you are always thinking about what you want, you will attract that "want." A clear goal was identified and written down. It was clear and concise. This act of contracting with his subconscious mind brought more power of imagination into his life. He went on to say if his career in show business didn't pan out, he would most likely be working in a steel mill in his hometown. He said the best jobs were in that mill. There is a quote by Sir John Hargrave, which states, "until it's on paper, its vapor."

Vignette 2
Where do you see yourself in 5 years?
In 5 years, I'd like to be the most valued nurse on your team. I plan to take full advantage of the continuing education reimbursement you offer to expand my skills beyond their current level. I'm skilled in patient education and electronic health record (EHR), which I know you value. There are so many new skills I'd like to gain, including budgeting and training others. I think my hospital is the perfect place to grow into a better nurse.

Vignette 3
Why is nursing rewarding to you?
For me, the rewards of nursing never stop coming. Every day I'm learning and growing in ways I never dreamed possible. I feel so good when I see my patients improve, and when I hold the hands of family members, providing emotional support in times of tragedy. Helping people feels better than anything else I've ever done, and I get paid for it! It's the most fantastic career I could imagine for myself.

References

Murphy M (2010) Hard goals: the secret to getting from where you are to where you want to be. McGraw-Hill Education, New York, NY

Patel (2020) 10 Powerful Ways to Master Self Discipline. Entrepreneur. https://www.entrepreneur.com/article/287005

The University of California, San Francisco (2020) Assess yourself -identifying your career development stage. https://career.ucsf.edu/assess-yourself-identifying-your-career-development-stage

Tips on Choosing the Right Nursing Job (n.d.). https://nurse.org/articles/choosing-the-right-nursing-job/

Building Your Career Path

RNs represent the largest segment of the US workforce and are among the highest-paid large occupations. There are more than 3.9 million registered nurses (RNs) in the USA. Among RNs working in the USA, 83% are actively employed in nursing. The majority (59.9%) of RNs work in hospitals. The average RN salary is $73,900 per year. RNs' positions are expected to grow from 2016 to 2026, which is faster than the average occupation. Most healthcare services involved nursing care in some way.

- References
- American Association of Colleges of Nursing (2020) Nursing fact sheet. https://www. aacnnursing.org/News-Information/Fact-Sheets/Nursing-Fact-Sheet
- Journal of Nursing Regulation (2018) The US nursing workforce in 2018 and beyond. https://www.journalofnursingregulation. com/article/S2155-8256(18)30015-2/full-text
- US Department of Health and Human Services (2018) National sample survey of registered nurses: brief summary of results. https://data.hrsa.gov/DataDownload/ NSSRN/GeneralPUF18/2018_NSSRN_Summary_Report-508.pdf

Contents

Professional Nursing Career Paths: The Non-academic Path

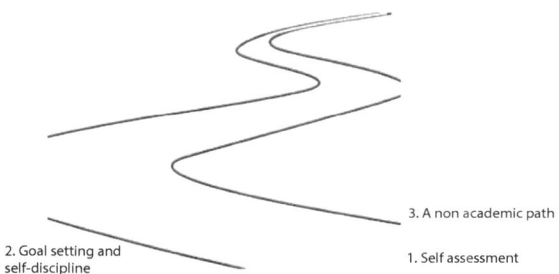

3. A non academic path

2. Goal setting and
self-discipline

1. Self assessment

Contents

© Springer Nature Switzerland AG 2020
J. M. Manning, *The Path to Building a Successful Nursing Career*,
https://doi.org/10.1007/978-3-030-50023-8_3

Rejoice in your work, never lose sight of the registered nurse (RN) you are now and the registered nurse (RN) you will become —Sue Fitzsimons

When you're a registered nurse (RN), you know that every day you will touch a life or a life will touch yours. —Unknown

The way to get started is to quit talking and begin doing. —Walt Disney

3.1 Introduction

The nursing profession encompasses a wide variety of career opportunities. These may range from entry-level practitioners to doctoral-level researchers. Many would add "it pays well too" and "they" would be correct. I caution you to think beyond the salary as you pursue your path and intentionally reflect on what you believe in and what you stand for. When you consider these additional factors, you will quickly see that your enthusiasm and passion will show, and success is likely to follow.

Nursing is a career and a professional choice. The consideration of nursing as an occupation or a career is crucial in understanding one's attitude towards nursing. An occupation is defined as an activity that keeps a person busy or a job. A career is a course of professional life that affords one with individual opportunities for personal advancement, progress, or achievement. Some view their nursing job as an occupation; others view it as a profession. The approach is essential to understand as this guides the nurse's attitude as possessing an "occupation" or a "career." Those who view nursing as a profession behave differently when compared to those who see it as a job or occupation (◘ Table 3.1).

A life choice must be planned and pursued. The obtaining of a nursing degree and a license is the ticket to get started. Without a goal and a map, the path may not be very long. A map with a plan will ensure milestones are met along the way, and opportunities are not missed. A map allows tracking of progress and ensures one stays on the path. Career management is the planned progression of one's professional life, which clearly defines goals.

3.2 Common Misconceptions in Nursing Careers

Good work in your nursing job will not serve to speak for itself. Quality patient care is the expectation of a nurse. It is commonly unnoticed until a mistake is made. Many nurses believe because of the ongoing nursing shortage, a job is guaranteed. A nursing shortage leads to the expansion of unlicensed personnel that are less qualified than a registered nurse (RN) and may erode the role of RNs. The belief a hospital will look out for the concerns of nurses is not realistic. Healthcare organizations are concerned with providing services to

3

◻ **Table 3.1**   Comparison of attitudes: nursing occupation vs. career

	Occupation	Career
Longevity	Temporary	Lifelong
Education	Minimal training, community college level	University-level training
Continuing Education	Complete what is required to maintain the job or to get a raise	Lifelong learners continually gain new knowledge, skills, and abilities
Commitment	Short term, based on job and personal needs	Long term, based on organization and profession
Expectation	Reasonable work for reasonable pay, responsibility ends with a shift	Assumes additional responsibilities, volunteers for organizational activities and community-based events

Masters, K. (2009) Role Development in Professional Nursing Practice. 5th ed. Jones and Bartlett.

patients for a cost. Nurses are one of the most expensive components of the economic equation, which hospitals must balance. Healthcare organizations operate in their own best interest, which may or may not align with nursing staff interests.

Nurses must take responsibility for managing their carers. One must seek a level of recognition and opportunities that will advance their career. Passive behavior will not lead you very far, and sitting back waiting for others to take care of your career is not their job, it is yours. You should not wait for good things to happen in your career; you must actively seek opportunities and make them happen to promote your best interest.

Case Example 3.1 Nursing Profession Common Myths

- ▬ If I work hard, rewards will come my way
- ▬ Excellent work by a nurse speaks for itself
- ▬ My boss needs to recommend me for advancement or promotion
- ▬ I am a nurse; I will always have a job
- ▬ My hospital is looking out for me and my best interests, always (Black 2016)

3.3 Certification

An investment in education should be guided by the long-term goals identified through reflection and self-assessment. An investment in education to obtain advanced certification is one strategy for those interested in advancing their career in the area of nursing management.

3.3.1 Benefits of Certification

When RNs certify, they expand their knowledge base in a particular area of specialty. Certification gives RNs the opportunity to advance their careers and prove their ability to provide the best patient care.

Certification benefits the RNs a career, patients, families, organizations, and the nursing profession. Certification provides validation that the registered nurse caring for them has demonstrated experience and knowledge in a complex specialty area. In today's dynamic healthcare environment, patients require heightened vigilance and high-level skills. Consumers are generally aware of the benefit of nursing certification. In a survey by the American Association of Critical Care Registered nurses (RNs) (AACN), it was reported 78% of participants knew RNs could be certified. Three in four stated they prefer to go to hospitals with RNs who are certified.

Certification of RNs benefits employers as well as RNs. Certified RNs are required to maintain ongoing continuing education (CE). Certification is a means for hospitals to differentiate themselves from the competition and demonstrate to the public they have the most skilled RN caring for their patients. Certification validates an ongoing high level of knowledge, experience, and skills. When employers support CE and certification, there is increased RN job satisfaction, which may result in a decreased likelihood of RN leaving their position or the hospitals. Employers play a crucial role in facilitating the decision for a RN to seek certification. When the employer promotes RN certification, they position themselves to thrive more competitively in the healthcare market. Through ongoing CE and experience, the RN becomes better at making an informed decision for the organization. Some malpractice companies offer discounts to certified RNs.

RN certification benefits RNs. RNs validate their knowledge and skills through certification. They position themselves for recognition, advancement, confidence, and achievement in their area of specialization. In some organizations, there is an increase in salary for certified RNs. Also, some organizations support the cost of certification exams, which removes the barrier of the cost associated with certifying. Certification validates specialty knowledge, experience, and clinical judgment. In 2010 study, RN's clinical judgment was validated through certification, and certified RNs reported that certification enabled them to experience personal growth and increase job satisfaction. As a voluntary process, certification emphasized the RN's commitment to career devilment and dedication to providing the highest level of patient care in a rapidly changing healthcare environment.

3

3.3.2 Descriptions of the Most Common RN Certifications

It is estimated there are nearly 200 nursing certification types! A list of nursing certifications can be found on registered nurse (RN).org (▶ https://registerednurse(RN).org/articles/nursing-certifications-credentials-list/). A 2015 survey reported 27% of RN respondents reported holding a certification. Among the younger population of RNs, 18% reported holding a certification. The largest area of certification was in Oncology (55%). Among ANCC Magnet recognized organizations, 37% of RNs report having certification (nursing world.org). You can easily identify which hospitals are Magnet recognized through a quick internet search on the American Registered Nurses (RNs) Credentialing Center (ANCC) website.

3.3.3 The Path to Successfully Certify in Nursing

The path to certification generally includes the following steps: determine eligibility for certification, apply for the certification, prepare for the exam, schedule the exam, take the exam, celebrate your certification, and learn about renewal steps. For in-depth information, refer to the specific certification exam of interest (◨ Fig. 3.1).

Many certification exams have handbooks that describe the test plan, testing details, sample questions, and references. Practice questions are an essential part of the preparation for the exam. Completion of self-assessment is a critical final step in preparation. Review courses are often used and can be very helpful in providing in-depth reviews by national experts. Review courses can be online or face to face. Typically, CE is available for those participating in review courses. Bookstores and online websites provide a wealth of information and references for certification preparation.

When reviewing for the exam, be sure to pay attention to the chapters which address the path for preparation. For example, when to start studying, how to study, etc. Also, if there is a chapter with strategies on controlling anxiety and how to handle answering questions you do not know, be sure to review with the same intensity as the chapters which address the content for the exam. For step 5, (◨ Fig. 3.1) ensure you are clear about testing locations, exam schedules, and responsibilities for the exam day. Also, ensure you review vital information for candidates with disabilities if you require accommodations during the exam.

3.4 Promotion

When an RN completes school and obtains a nursing license, they are a generalist. Once they begin employment, they are part of a system that has many specialized areas. Many of these areas employ RNs to work in specialized roles. Over time, many RNs will find a niche or passion for a specific area of practice. For example,

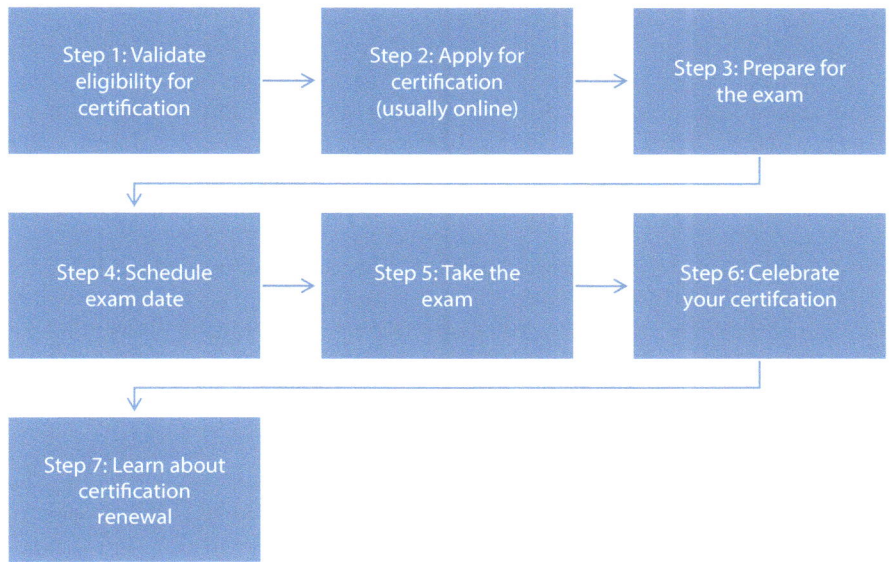

◘ Fig. 3.1 Steps to nursing certification (American Association of Critical-Care Nurses 2020)

some RNs may find a niche in a particular type of patient care areas such as women's health, oncology, or critical care. Some may find a niche with a particular kind of patient, older patients such as in geriatrics or younger patients such as with pediatrics. A RN may find a niche with a type of patient care areas such as surgery or an outpatient clinic.

At some point, there may be an interest in moving up or getting promoted. One may ask how to get there? You may look at someone else and wonder what did this person do to get where they are? I encourage you never to be afraid to ask that person these questions. Offer to buy that person coffee and ask for 15 minutes of their time. Bring a list of critical questions you want to ask and let them talk. Their stories are typically entertaining, and their path is rarely a straight one where there were several twists and turns. You may find that you are encouraged by the fact that the path wasn't straightforward nor always easy to accomplish.

There are many ways to increase your likelihood of getting promoted in nursing. They include:

1. **Stay motivated with your career development plan**

Staying motivated requires optimism and commitment. Your goals must be at the forefront of your mind, and you should reward the "small victories."

2. **Enjoy your job, be passionate**

When you think of your job, consider what your job allows you to have in your life. Keep a positive attitude. Nurses are consistently positively viewed in the public. They have a reputation of being honest, caring, reliable, concerned, caring, and

3

approachable. They are part of a prestigious profession. Plan your time and create a to-do list. Focus on the tasks at hand in your work. Ensure you are clear about your expectations and delegate when applicable. Be sure to take breaks regularly. Relax at work and promote a pleasant work environment. Reflect on your day and how you can make improvements. Ensure you have downtime at home to recharge and reflect.

3. Keep learning and be a resource to others

Stay up to date in the work environment. Know the priorities and what is the current quality improvement projects. Read literature in nursing as well as outside of nursing. Discuss the issues with others in the work environment. Remember, when discussing problems, also end with a focus on potential solutions. Otherwise, you are just wining, which is nonproductive.

4. Be a team player

Show others you are committed to the team. Be as flexible as possible. Be reliable and responsible. Listen to others. Keep others informed of what is going on. Always be willing to help another—support and respect others.

5. Find a mentor

» Successful people never reach their goals alone – Glenn Hole

Mentors expose you to new ideas and ways of thinking. They offer advice on developing strengths and overcoming weaknesses. Mentors are a great source of information on career development. One should identify experienced and successful people they are comfortable with inside and outside of your organization. Do not be afraid to ask for career guidance and advice from someone with more experience than you.

6. Be a mentor

While you may not realize if you have much to contribute, no matter where you are in your career, there is always someone who would benefit from hearing your story and how you got where you are. Even if you are not finished your career journey, be a mentor to them, offer accurate information, and show interest in their success.

7. Learn to ask for things you want

Many people are very good at expressing what makes them unhappy or how they may have been "wronged" by someone. They are not very good at following up on the problem they are facing with a solution or a statement of what they want. Learning to strategically express a problem or situation and following up with a suggestion on how to improve the situation or solve the problem is essential in moving forward. Be sure you are asking for what you want. Consider the context of the situation, the timing, the person you are talking to, the big picture, and their perspective.

◘ Table 3.2 Eight key organizational characteristics

Philosophy	Does the employer exemplify a philosophy of clinical care based on quality, safety, interdisciplinary collaboration, continuity of care, and professional accountability?
Value	Does the employer recognize the importance of nurses' expertise in clinical care quality and patient outcomes?
Leadership	Does the employer promote executive level leadership in nursing?
Empowerment	Does the employer empower nurses participation in clinical decision-making and organization of local care systems
Professional Development	Does the employer support professional development for nurses?
Clinical Advancement Programs	Does the employer maintain clinical advancement programs based on education, certification, and preparation?
Collaborate	Does the employer create collaborative relationships among healthcare team members?
Technology	Do employers use technological advances in clinical care and information systems?

American Nurses Credentialing Center (2020)

ANCC describes eight critical characteristics for a nurse to consider when screening a potential employer (◘ Table 3.2).

8. Do not keep your head down and hope for the best

When searching for the right position, use technology to help you identify the most current job posting. Review the organization's mission and philosophy. Do they align with your values and beliefs? Review the description of the facility, the services they offer. Contact a person in the area who may be familiar with the organization. Ask their opinion about the organization. Contact the organization. Remember, first impressions are essential.

■ **You must actively search for what you want**

Look at your goals frequently, revise them as needed. Be proactive in your search to advance your career. Ensure you are positioning yourself for the opportunity. Are you participating in organizational activities, talking to others about opportunities, revising the job postings for opportunities you may want to secure? You need to position yourself through visibility, competency, and passion.

3

■ **Career development is more than showing up for work and doing your job**

It involves a commitment to your work. Your efforts must go beyond the care of patients on your unit to responsibilities beyond those for which you were hired. Administering high-quality patient care is only one part of the nurse's role. If you aim to advance your career, you must be seen as a committed member of the organization who aligns with organizational goals. You must be visible.

■ **Good work does not speak for itself**

Nurses who show up on time, do a good job, and go home are rarely recognized by the influential people in the organization unless a problem occurs. Night shift nurses are even less known and seldom seen by the administration. They run the risk of being invisible to the organization if they do not engage in activities that occur during regular business hours. How to increase visibility?

■ **Self-governance and committee work**

Hospitals are led by governance structure and committee work. Hospital committee examples include ethics committees, research committees, patient care committees, quality committees, audit committees, protocol review committees, etc. Volunteering to serve contributes to your professional autonomy and provides opportunities for others to see you in a different light and how you're helpful to the organization. Most healthcare organizations participate in blood drives, fundraising, and health fairs. These opportunities allow nurses to give back to the community while getting to know people in other areas of the organization.
━ Competency and Improving Skills

Nursing is a lifelong career of learning. You must remain competent and build your competence. Nurses have the privilege of interacting with people during the most critical moments of their lives—birth, death, illness, and injury. The work of nurses impacts the lives of others when they are the most vulnerable and in need— the work of nurses matters and actions count. You need to ensure others know what you are doing to keep your skills current and developing new skills. Do not keep these a secret. Create a resume that is current and well developed. Use these tips for preparing your resume (◼ Table 3.3):
━ Culture/professionalism

Professionalism must always be upheld. Understand others are watching you (not in a creepy way!) and considering whether your behaviors should be role modeled. As an RN, our professionalism defines us and guides our future development.

Whatever practice level or desired specialty, a certification in nursing is out there for you to achieve. Through certification, you demonstrate exceptional expertise in a specialized area with continuing competency.

3.5 Nursing Specialties

》 There is nothing as useless as doing efficiently that which should not be done at all

◘ Table 3.3 Tips for resume preparation

Resume Essentials	Begin your resume with your aim Include a self-assessment of your 　Skills 　Abilities 　Education 　Work experience 　Extracurricular activities
Content of Resume	Include *Contact information*—name, address, phone, email and credentials 　Do not include nicknames 　Use a permanent address and phone number with area code 　Ensure you have a neutral greeting on your voicemail 　Provide a professional email address *Objective* 　State the work you seek to find 　Be specific 　Tailor your objective for each employer, no generic objectives *Education* 　New graduates without work experience should list education information first 　List most recent education first, end with the last (reverse chronological order) 　Include degree, major, institution attended, major and minor concentrations 　Add GPA if more than 3.0 　Mention any academic honors (scholarship/grant, awards, dean list, honor societies, recognitions) *Work Experience* 　Provide a brief overview of work that has taught you skills 　Use action verbs to describe job duties 　List in reverse chronological order 　Include the title of position, name of the organization, location (city and state), dates of employment, work responsibilities, skills and achievements 　Other 　Include special skills or key competencies 　Leadership experience in organizations (include volunteer) 　Participation in sports 　References 　Ask people if they will serve as a reference before giving their name to an employer 　Do not list names and addresses of references. Note "references furnished on request" at the bottom of resume and provide when requested 　Final check 　Proofread for spelling and grammar errors If you are sending via post office mail: 　Print on plain quality bond paper 　Single side only 　12 to 14 font 　Avoid decorative embellishments 　Do not fold or staple 　If mailing, place in a large envelope

McGrimmon (2013)

3

» The difficulty lies not in the new ideas but in escaping the old ones

As healthcare has become more sophisticated, RNs are finding new nontraditional roles away from the bedside and into community-based settings. Nursing is a career with a tremendous variety of roles and career options. Regardless of your starting point in your career, there are opportunities in many areas.

RNs can play key roles in specialized patient care areas. In each of these areas, certification can be obtained to demonstrate expertise. Not all nurses work at the bedside for their entire career. You may find yourself looking for a change of pace or wanting to use your skills in another way away from the bedside. There are many nursing specialty areas. The following sections include a list of potential specialty areas. This list does not include all nursing speciality areas currently available.

3.5.1 Ambulatory Care Nurse

An ambulatory care nurse provides care to patients in non-emergency situations in outpatient care environments. Ambulatory care nurses work directly with patients. This type of nurse can work on their own or start a practice. The scope of the practice will depend on the state rules and regulations for RNs. The American Academy of Ambulatory Care Nursing is a helpful resource for gaining information in this field.

3.5.2 Burn Care Nurse

A burn care nurse provides care to patients who have been burned by fire, chemicals, electricity, hot water, or oil. They work directly with patients. They provide care to burn patients and their families and educate the community regarding burn prevention. The burn care nurse has expertise in stabilizing burns, dressing, and caring for wounds and medication administration. They work in hospital settings in burn care units, emergency rooms, trauma centers, and intensive care units. The American Burn Association and Burn Nurse Practitioner are both helpful resources for gaining information in this field.

3.5.3 Camp Nurse

Camp nurses care for people attending camps or retreats, which are typically located far from hospitals. They work with patients directly. They may lead, guide, and support nurses in providing camp care. They educate campers in burn prevention, outdoor safety, etc. They administer first aid and medications to campers, attendees, and staff participating in the camp. They participate in pre-camp assessments, document camper visits, and maintain first aid supplies for the camp. The Association of Camp Nursing (ACN) is a great place to learn more about camp nursing.

3.5.4 **Cardiac Care Nurse**

Cardiac care nurses care for patients with heart disease or conditions from heart failure, bypass surgery, or coronary heart disease. Cardiac care nurses work with patients and cardiologists. They perform stress tests, monitor heart activity, and electrocardiograms. They administer medications, monitor pain, and manage intravenous lines. They teach patients and families about heart disease, treatments, and preventative heart care.

Cardiac care nurses may work in hospitals but also clinics, nursing homes, and home health. A cardiac cath lab nurse is a type of cardiac care nurse who works with patients who have catheters inserted into their hearts to evaluate cardiac conditions or heart defects. Cath lab nurses work with a cardiologist in providing care to patients. They administer medications and monitor patients. They teach patients about heart disease and how to prevent the worsening of their heart condition. The Preventative Cardiovascular Nurses Association, American Association of Heart Failure Nurses, and Council on Cardiovascular and Stroke Nursing are all helpful resources for gaining information in this field.

3.5.5 **Case Management Nurse**

RN case managers coordinate the various components of patient care. They maximize the use of resources and services for patients. They work between different healthcare environments, such as inpatient and outpatient settings. Case managers screen, assess, determine risk, plan, implement, follow up, transition, communicate, and evaluate the care needed to ensure optimal patient outcomes. RNs can obtain certification in case management. For example, they can become a certified case manager (CCM). The American Case Management Association, Case Management Society of America, the American Association Managed Care Nurses, American Academy of Case Management are all helpful resources for gaining information in this field (Johnson and Johnson 2020).

3.5.6 **Critical Care RN (CCRN)**

Critical care RN (CCRN) treats patients with acute and sometimes life-threatening injuries. They have specialized knowledge in monitoring patients who are seriously ill or injured. The American Association of Critical Care Nurses, Critical Care, and Emergency Nurses Association are both helpful resources for gaining information in this field.

3

3.5.7 Dialysis RN

A dialysis RN (CCRN) works in the area of nephrology and has specialized knowledge regarding kidney disease. They provide care to patients who receive dialysis by giving support, medications, and monitoring. They educate patients regarding kidney disease management. The American Nephrology Nurses Association is a great resource for gaining information in this field.

3.5.8 Geriatric RN

A geriatric RN, also called gerontological RN, cares for older adult (greater than 65 years old) clients. They have specialized education in the care of older adult (greater than 65 years old) patients. They help patients recover from illness or injury. They may assist with rehabilitation and conduct patient care visits in skilled care or hospice facilities. The Coalition of Geriatric Nursing Organizations, Gerontological Advanced Practice Nurses Association, American Geriatrics Society, and National Gerontological Nursing Association are all helpful resources for gaining information in this field.

3.5.9 Health and Wellness RN Coach

A health and wellness RN coach facilitates behavior changes. This type of RN may be called "wellness RN" who monitors the health of patients. Much of their role is in education to empower patients to optimize self-care. RNs may work with older adults or patients with chronic health issues. There is a health coach certification RNs can obtain, such as Health and Wellness Registered nurse (RN) Coach Board Certified (HWNC-BC). The American Holistic Nurses Association is a helpful resource for gaining information in this field.

3.5.10 Health Policy RN

A health policy RN works in the planning, policy, and management of healthcare. They play a pivotal role in improving the quality and safety of care. Their role may include analyzing and evaluating healthcare policies, laws, or regulations. The unique perspective of an RN offers the health policy RN an opportunity to lead as a healthcare change agent. Policy decides who receives funds, the amount, and for what programs. RNs have much to contribute in this area. In this role, an RN may be responsible for a variety of government affairs operations, advocacy, and organizational policy. The role includes moving issues forward, collaboration, discussion, and debate on relevant policies. In this role, an RN can speak up for patients and populations by offering crucial information about the healthcare systems. The American Nurses Association and American Academy of Nursing are both helpful resources for gaining knowledge in this field.

3.5.11   Hospice RN

A hospice RN is a nursing specialty where the nurse is trained to work closely with patients at the end of life. Hospice nurses play a role as a case manager and patient advocate. They work closely with families. The work of a hospice nurse is emotional, and specialized training is needed to ensure nurses are prepared to work in this type of patient care setting. Hospice nurses work in hospice clinics or patient homes. The focus is on helping patients live comfortably as they near and at the end of life. Patient care includes pain management and vital sign monitoring. Nurses may take on additional roles as needed for the unique patient care needs, such as ensuring supplies are provided to patients. They facilitate coping and provide support to families and significant others. In addition to being an RN, a hospice nurse can choose to certify through the National Board for certification of hospice and palliative nurses. Certification requires experience in hospice settings. The Hospice and Palliative Nurses Association, National Hospice and Palliative Care Organization, and the American Nurses Association are all helpful resources for gaining information in this field.

3.5.12   Informatics RNs

Nursing informatics is a field of nursing which incorporates information sciences and nursing to manage and develop medical data. Through this work, an informatics RN can support nursing practice and improve patient outcomes. RN informaticists develop communication and information technology in healthcare. They can serve as educators, researchers, or software engineers. They establish policies and procedures for organizations.

An informatics RN focuses on the management of information and communication. This type of RN facilitates data integration, information knowledge to best support patients, RNs, and healthcare providers. Skills in computers and data systems are needed to improve patient care outcomes. This field is growing with an estimate of more than 70,000 nursing informatics specialists anticipated to be required by 2025. The American Nursing Informatics Association and Alliance for Nursing Informatics are both helpful resources for information on this field of nursing.

▶ https://nursejournal.org/nursing-informatics/nursing-informatics-career-outlook/

3.5.13   Lactation Consultant

A lactation consultant is a breastfeeding specialist who trains moms on feeding their babies. They assist women with breastfeeding problems such as latching difficulties, painful breastfeeding, and diminished milk production. They help with babies who are aren't gaining weight.

The United States Lactation Consultant Association and International Lactation Consultant Association are both helpful resources for information on this field of nursing.

3.5.14 Legal RN Consultant

A legal nurse consultant (LNC) combines their expertise as a healthcare provider in consulting on medical-related legal cases. LNCs assist attorneys in reviewing medical records and understanding healthcare issues to achieve the best results for their clients. They help with the understanding of medical terminology and scope of practice. Typically, a LNC bridges a gap between an attorney's knowledge of the legal system and the healthcare system. LNCs may screen a case for merit, assist with discovery, conduct literature reviews, review medical records, and clarify standards of care. They may prepare reports or summarize the extent of a client's injury or illness.

The LNC is a member of the legal team, often providing critical information for the case. An LNC is a certified RN, and legal education is not a requirement. LNCs work for legal firms, government agencies, insurance companies, and hospital risk management departments. They may be self-employed. There are a variety of training programs, and while there are several certification types. The American Legal Registered nurse (RN) Consultation Certification Board offers one certification exam. The American Association of Legal Nurse Consultants and the National Alliance of Certified Legal Nurse Consultants are both helpful resources for information on this field of nursing.

3.5.15 Occupational RN

An occupational health nurse (OHN) provides and delivers health and safety programs to worker populations or community groups. The emphasis is on promotion, restoration, or maintenance of health, prevention of illness and injury from environmental hazards. OHNs combine knowledge of health and business to ensure balance in the work environment. An RN can become a certified occupational health RN (COHN). The American Association of Occupational Health Nurses is a helpful resource for information on this field of nursing.

3.5.16 Pain Management RN

Pain management RN assess patients to determine the cause of their pain and severity. They may administer medications or teach patients how to manage their medications. They may introduce patients to alternative pain management techniques. The American Society for Pain Management Nursing and American Chronic Pain Association are both helpful resources for information on this field of nursing.

3.5.17 Pediatric RN

A pediatric RN works in preventative and acute care settings with children and adolescents. They provide education and support patient families. They may go on to become APRNs and assess, diagnose pediatric clients. The Society of Pediatric Nursing Associations and the National Association of Pediatric Nurse Practitioners are helpful resources for obtaining information on this field of nursing. Additionally, there are many specialized pediatric nurse associations such as the Association of Pediatric Hematology-Oncology Nurses and the American Pediatric Surgical Nurses Association.

3.5.18 Psychiatric RN

A psychiatric-mental health RN works with individuals, families, and groups in assessing mental health needs. They may go on to become an APRN in this field, which includes further training in assessing, diagnosing, and treating individuals with psychiatric disorders or identify risk factors for developing diseases. The American Psychiatric Nurses Association and International Society of Psychiatric-Mental Health Nurses are both helpful resources for information on this field of nursing.

3.5.19 Public Health Nursing

A public health RN works to improve the health of communities and improve care access. They typically work with patients in communities. Public health RNs have the potential to make significant differences in the protection of population health. Through their health knowledge, they influence the health and wellbeing of patients. The public health RN encourages lifestyle changes in the community and offers education to some of the most vulnerable populations. An RN can become a certified public health RN (PHN). The Association of Public Health Nurses and Quad Council Coalition of Public Health Nursing Organizations are both helpful resources for information on this field of nursing.

3.5.20 Quality Nursing

A quality RN supports clinical bedside RNs in meeting regulatory measures, which ultimately impacts patient outcomes. Another name for quality RN is utilization review RN. Quality RNs work behind the scenes to ensure quality care is maximized and cost-efficient. Quality RNs can assist patients in making informed decisions about their healthcare and educate them on the benefits and limitations of their insurance. RNs can obtain several different types of quality certifications. For example, they can become a certified professional in healthcare quality (CPHQ). The ANA Nursing Alliance for Quality Care and National Association for Healthcare Quality are both helpful resources for information on this field of nursing.

3

3.5.21   RN Author

An RN writer, or author, contributes educational material, historical books, movie/television scripts about nursing in the written form. This style of nursing is much different from the bedside, and the registered nurse (RN) uses pen/paper instead of a stethoscope. Many registered nurse (RN) writers work freelance. They apply nursing skills to writing. They educate others in nursing work and healthcare. The American Medical Writers Association and ANA are helpful resources for information on this field of nursing.

3.5.22   RN Educators

An RN educator trains the next generation of registered nurses (RNs). Registered nurse (RN) educators are essential for ensuring the RN workforce can meet the healthcare needs of current and future generations. Colleges are faced with pressure to find qualified faculty to educate the future nursing workforce due to non-competitive salaries with clinical positions. Registered nurse (RN) educators serve an essential role within the hospital system. Nurse educator knowledge and experience in their field of expertise is passed on to student nurses in their training. Clinical nurse educators (CNE) are similarly training registered nurses in a specialized field of nursing to improve patient care and hospital outcomes. The National League for Nursing, nurse educator resource center, professional nurse educator group, and American Association of Colleges of Nursing are all helpful resources for gaining information on this field of nursing (◘ Figs. 3.2 and 3.3).

3.5.23   RN Executive

RN executives lead the management and administrative side of patient care services. They collaborate with other health professionals, develop partnerships and networks. RN executives play a key role in the healthcare system. They oversee the achievement of organizational goals. They lead, guide, and support RNs by supporting their ability to provide quality patient care. RN executives need to possess skills in budgeting, communication, and organizational policy management. The American Organization for Nursing Leadership and Organization of Nurse Leaders are both helpful resources for gaining information in this field.

3.5.24   RN Manager

RN managers supervise nursing staff in clinical settings. RN managers have many duties. They include staff management, case management, recruitment, budgeting, scheduling, and mentoring. The American Organization for Nursing Leadership is a helpful resource for gaining information in this field.

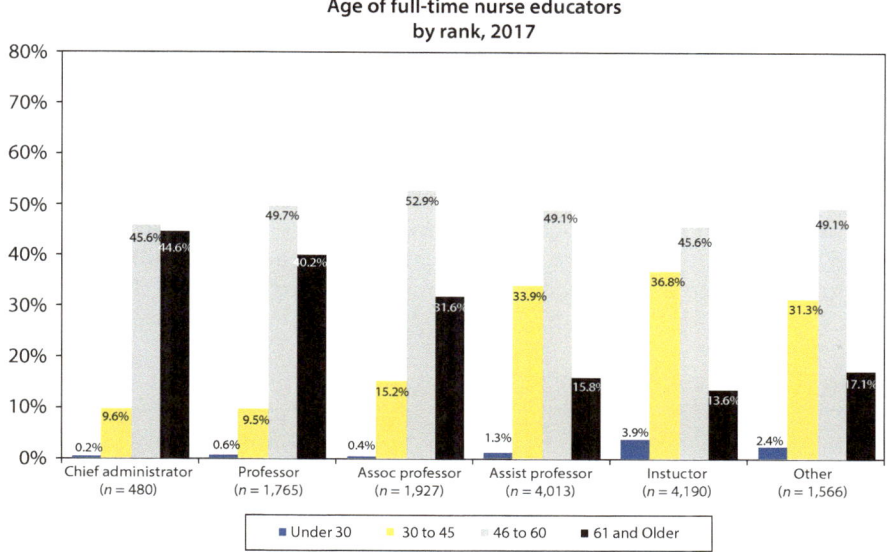

● **Fig. 3.2**   Age of full-time nurse educators (National League for Nursing 2018a)

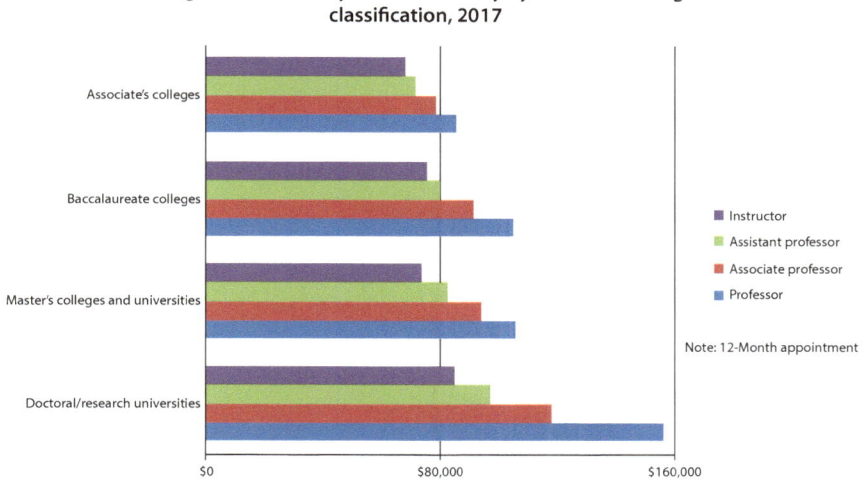

● **Fig. 3.3**   Average full-time salary for nurse faculty (National League for Nursing 2018b)

3

3.5.25 RN Researchers

An RN researcher applies nursing skills in commercial and academic research. They work in universities, pharmaceutical companies, hospitals, and other settings. RN researchers study various aspects of health, illness, and healthcare. They design and carry out studies that aim to improve health, healthcare services, and health outcomes. They publish research and disseminate findings in local, national, and international settings. The International Association of Clinical Research Nurses, the National Institute of Nursing Research, and the Association of Clinical Research Professionals are all helpful in obtaining information on this field.

3.5.26 Trauma RN

A trauma RN manages minor and acute patient care problems. They may prepare patients for emergency surgery or assist surgeons in surgery. They help patients with severe injuries such as myocardial infarction, stroke, attempted suicide, motor vehicle accidents, or other injuries. The Society of Trauma Nurses and Emergency Nurses Association are both helpful in obtaining information on this field.

3.5.27 Travel RN

A travel RN works based on a contract, typically more than 10 weeks to fill a hospital's needs. They work in temporary positions, most commonly in hospital settings. Nurses go to places where their specialties and skills are in demand. Typically, travel staffing companies include pay packages that take care of the nurse's housing costs, meals, and incidental expenditures. Nurses can travel domestically or internationally. The adventure of travel nursing is appealing as the nurse experiences new people and new places. Depending on where a nurse travels, more money can be made. Also, nurses avoid payroll taxes because they qualify for tax-free stipends. Travel nurses can grow professionally by experiencing different hospitals and developing a broad range of skills.

There are some considerations for travel nursing. The nurse is away from their home state and away from family and friends. The nurse moves around a lot. If the nurse uses their vehicle, they will put a lot of mileage on it. They search for new contracts frequently, as often as every 3 months, which can be time-consuming. There is always the risk of a cancellation of the contract, and the paperwork can be daunting. Typically the orientation is abbreviated, and the nurse must acclimate to the new work environment quickly. The American Travel Health Nurses Association and National Association of Travel Healthcare Organizations are both helpful in obtaining information on this field.

Many of these specialty areas have existed for some time. As healthcare changes, new certification areas are emerging.

Strategies

Take this quiz to explore what type of RN you should be.

Gotoquiz.com has a quiz that helps a person decide which area of nursing may be best for them. After completing the questionnaire, feedback is provided based on responses. ► https://www.gotoquiz.com/what_nursing_specialty_are_you

Johnson and Johnson offers an online questionnaire to facilitate the finding of a nrusing specialty. Suggestions are provided based on respones. ► https://nursing.jnj.com/find-my-specialty/

❓ Activities

Consider your personality traits and the kind of person you are. The best nursing career path for you is one that best matches your personality and aptitude. For example, do you like working with older adults, then gerontology may be the field for you. Do you like working with children? Then pediatrics may be the field for you. Do you want a fast-paced, challenging environment? Then critical care may be for you. Often RNs ask, "what type of nursing specialty is for me?"

Several online quizzes are available for free to help with exploring nursing areas which are a good match for you. Beyond an online questionnaire, you should connect with an RN who is working in the field you are interested in. Ask to meet with them. Develop a list of questions to ask them. Visit their work environment. Possibly shadow them for a day. All of this work will pay off, in the end, to ensure you pursue a career match that is best for you.

► https://www.quizony.com/what-kind-of-registerednurse(RN)-should-i-be/index.html

► https://www.herzing.edu/blog/which-nursing-specialty-right-you

Vignettes
Vignette 1

Question: Why did you pursue advanced education in nursing?

After completing my BSN, I found myself in a medical-surgical unit, where I learned how to be an RN. I cherished every day, worked hard, and delivered excellent nursing care with the guidance of a mentor. Over time I found myself asking more and more questions, such as why do we chart bowel movements in 3 places, is this necessary? The answer I received was, "we have always done it that way." Finding little satisfaction in those responses, I decided my career would not continue in medical-surgical unit nursing. I moved on to a critical care unit and moved to the night shift 2 years later. I was again challenged and enjoyed the new experience. I learned new things and enjoyed still working hard and providing excellent nursing care. I again found myself asking the same questions with the same response. I decided to try for a master's degree (there were no DNP programs at that time). I went to school during the day and worked

3

nights. I graduated with my APRN and moved on to a place where I could autonomously make decisions. I did not want to keep doing things "the same way we have always done it." I put myself in a position where I had the knowledge and confidence to make larger-scale changes in the hospital.

Vignette 2

What do you find most challenging about being a nurse?

I think the most challenging part of being a nurse is when I have a patient that is very unhappy or is in a lot of pain, and I can't comfort them to the degree I'd like to. I keep a dialog going with the attending physician so that he has as much information as possible regarding the patient's pain level. Sometimes the patient doesn't effectively communicate with the doctor, and I try to help bridge that communication gap.

Vignette 3

Why did you choose to become a nurse?

Nurses have such an influential role in the hospital. I saw that first-hand when I was young and had a family member in the hospital, and it made me determined to pursue the career. Helping people during a difficult time is tremendously meaningful to me.

Vignette 4

Jenny is a 23-year-old RN who graduated from an associated degree program four years ago. She has worked at a large hospital in a major city. She began her career in an oncology unit and transferred to a cardiology unit. She is an outstanding nurse and provides excellent care to patients. She is a team player in her unit and has had positive evaluations. She wants to go back to school for her BSN. She faces many challenges, the cost of school, juggling shift work, and family obligations. An opening on her unit became available recently for the assistant nurse manager position. She was not considered and was disappointed when a less experienced colleague accepted the position. Jenny asked her manager why she was not recognized. Her manager told Jenny she did not know she was interested. Jenny felt devalued.

This story is commonly the way nurses approach their jobs. Career development is not a familiar concept to them, and they see nursing as "a calling." Many see advancement in their positions as "self-promotion." They are uncomfortable in calling attention to their accomplishments and do not ask for raises, promotions, or recognition. The result is a lack of positive feedback, career advancement opportunities, and recognition. Nurses who feel stagnant in their careers may become burned out, change jobs, or leave the nursing practice.

References

American Association of Critical-Care Nurses (2020) Certification benefits patients, employers, and nurses. Retrieved from: https://www.aacn.org/certification/value-of-certification-resource-center/registered nurse (RN)-certification-benefits-patients-employers-and-registered nurse (RN)s

American Nurses Credentialing Center (2020) Facts about the Magnet Recognition Program. Retrieved from: https://www.nursingworld.org/globalassets/organizational-programs/magnet/magnet-factsheet.pdf

Black B (2016) Professional nursing, 8th edn. Elsevier

Johnson and Johnson (2020) Find a specialty. Retrieved from: https://nursing.jnj.com/specialty

McGrimmon L (2013) The resume writing guide: a step by step workbook for creating a winning resume, 2nd edn. CareerChoiceGuide

National League for Nursing (2018a) Faculty census survey. Retrieved from: http://www.nln.org/docs/default-source/default-document-library/age-of-full-time-nurse-educators-by-rank-2017.pdf?sfvrsn=0

National League for Nursing (2018b) Faculty census survey. Retrieved from: http://www.nln.org/docs/default-source/default-document-library/average-full-time-salary-of-nurse-educators-on-12-month-appointment-by-rank-and-carnegie-classification-2017.pdf?sfvrsn=0

Professional Nursing Career Paths: The Academic Path

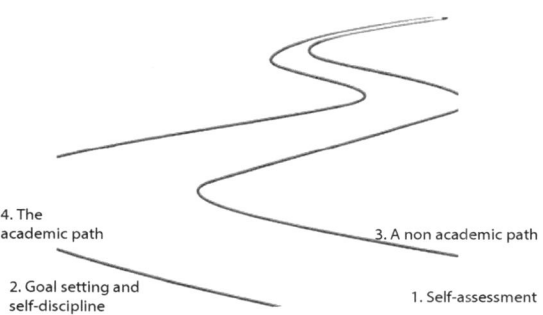

Contents

© Springer Nature Switzerland AG 2020
J. M. Manning, *The Path to Building a Successful Nursing Career*,
https://doi.org/10.1007/978-3-030-50023-8_4

Education is the key to unlocking the world, a passport to freedom. —Oprah Winfrey

4.1 Introduction

In 2018, there were 2.8 million registered nurses (RNs) and 690,000 licensed practical nurses (LPN) in the United States. The majority of RNs are female (91%) over a wide variety of age ranges (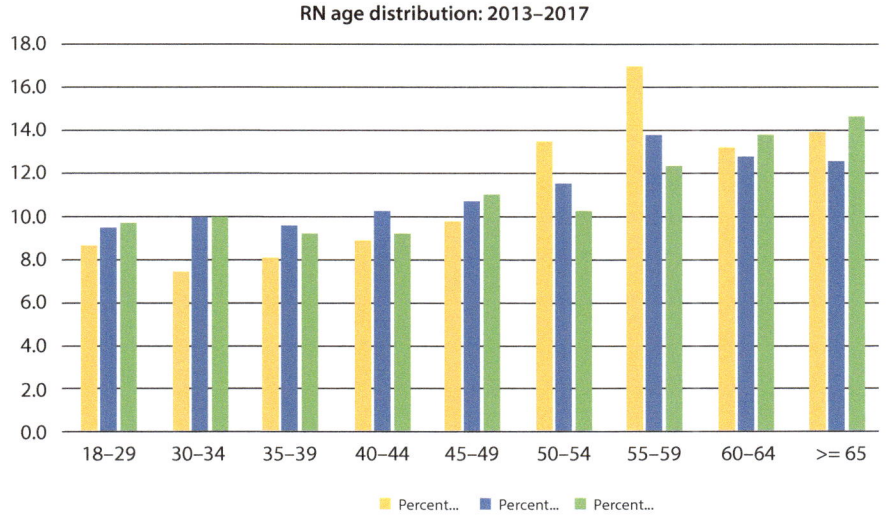 Figs. 4.1 and 4.2). Considering ethnic backgrounds, 80% of RNs are White, 6.2% African American, 7.5% Asian, 5.3 Hispanic, 0.4% American Indian/Alaskan Native, and 0.5% Native Hawaiian/Pacific Islander (■ Fig 4.3). Forty four percent of RNs held a bachelor's degree, and 19.3% held a graduate degree (■ Fig 4.4). Among those with a graduate degree, 17% of RNs held a master's degree and 1.9% a doctoral degree.

The demand for more highly educated registered nurses (RNs) far outweighs the supply (American Association of Colleges of Nursing (2020a)).

There are several levels of nursing degrees. If you are confused by the levels of nursing education, you are not alone. The title of "registered nurse (RN)" is used to describe many groups, which results in confusion among the public, professionals, and organizations. It is crucial to understand the differences among the various "nursing roles" when on your path to build a successful nursing career.

Furthering your career through education and going to school will advance your nursing career. Education improves your nursing knowledge and skills, which

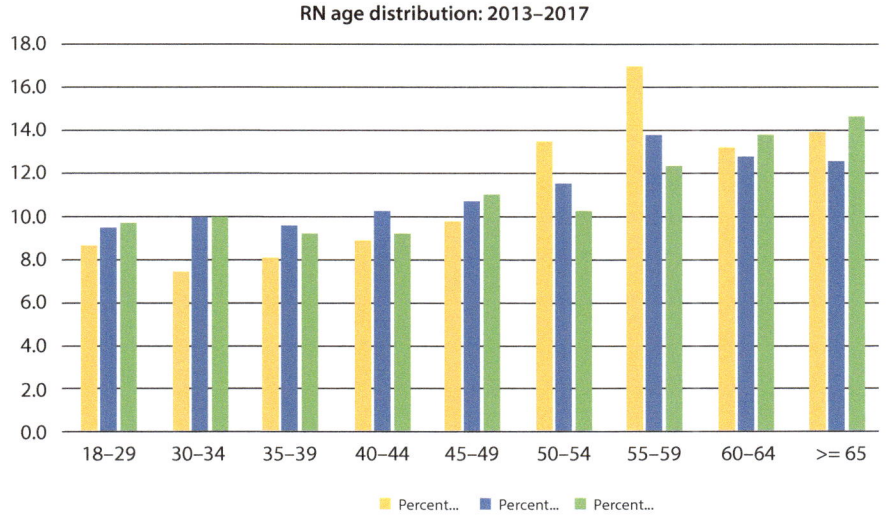

■ **Fig. 4.1**   RN age distribution (National Councils for State Boards of Nursing 2020)

4

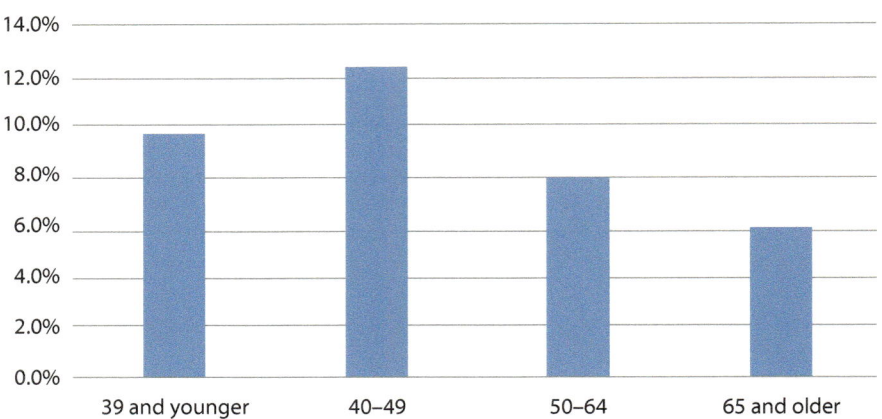

Fig. 4.2 Percent of RNs who are male and percent of RNs who are male by age group (National Councils for State Boards of Nursing 2020)

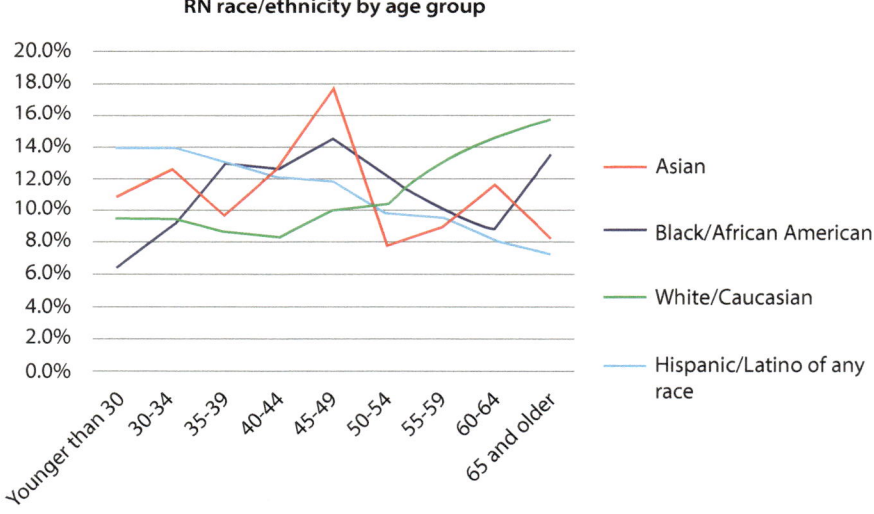

Fig. 4.3 RN race by age group (National Councils for State Boards of Nursing 2020)

can lead to a nursing career or further advancement in your career. Educational programs provide you with the tools and credentials you need to achieve your career goals (Fitzpatrick 2017). CNAs and LPNs work under the supervision of an RN. An RN can possess a diploma, Associates Degree or a Bachelors Degree (■ Fig. 4.5).

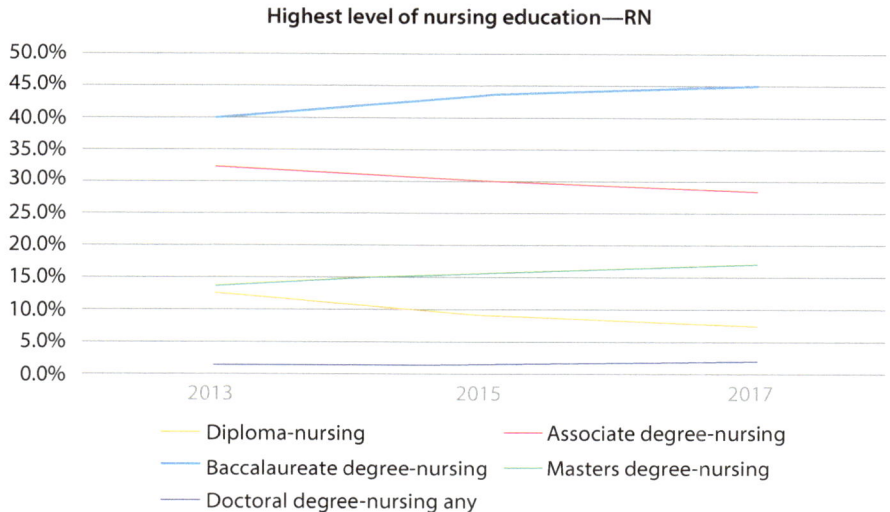

Fig. 4.4 Highest level of nursing education (National Councils for State Boards of Nursing 2020)

Fig. 4.5 Types of registered nursing degrees

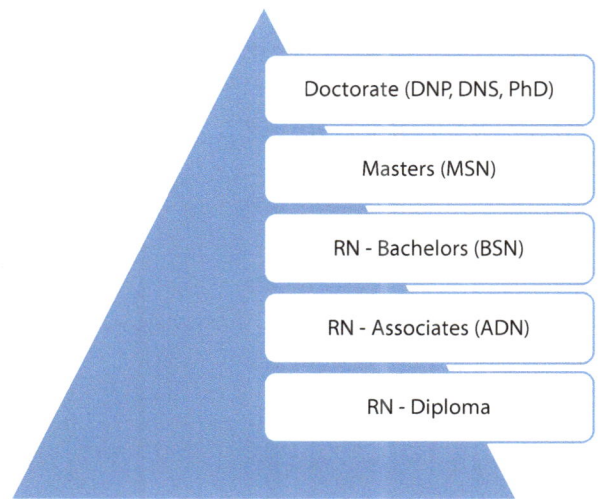

4.2 Certified Nursing Assistant (CNA)

A certified nursing assistant provides basic care to patients. Students typically complete their program in 12 weeks through a combination of classroom instruction and clinical training. CNAs assist patients with daily activities, take vital signs, set up medical equipment, and assist with medical procedures.

4.3 Licensed Practical Nurse (LPN)

The LPN prepares a nurse to perform nursing duties. Students typically complete their program in 1 year through a combination of classroom instruction and clinical training. The LPN can obtain their degree through a diploma-based program or an associate's degree program. Programs are typically offered through community colleges. LPNs are employed in many settings, including long-term care facilities where they provide direct nursing care, usually led by an RN. This degree is a fast way to enter the nursing field. The scope of work is limited, and you may be faced with going back to school to expand more opportunities. It is essential to look into both the LPN and RN option before deciding your path as it is not always cheaper and faster than becoming an RN. Also, salary growth, as well as career opportunities, may not be as expansive.

The types of nursing degrees include diploma, an associate degree in nursing (ADN), Bachelor of Science in Nursing (BSN, Master of Science in Nursing (MSN), and Doctor of Nursing (Ph.D., DNP, DNS) (☒ Fig. 4.5).

4.4 Registered Nurse (RN)

A registered nurse (RN) can coordinate patient care, educate patients and the public about health conditions. RNs provide emotional support to patients and family members. They are not limited in the scope of medication administration like LPNs. To take the National Council Licensure Examination (NCLEX) exam, a student must graduate from a Diploma program, Associates, or Bachelor degree nursing program (☒ Figs. 4.6, 4.7, and 4.8). Growth of the profession is increasing and nurses earn some of the highest salaries in healthcare (☒ Fig. 4.6). RNs work across a wide variety of settings (☒ Fig 4.7) and specialties (☒ Fig. 4.8).

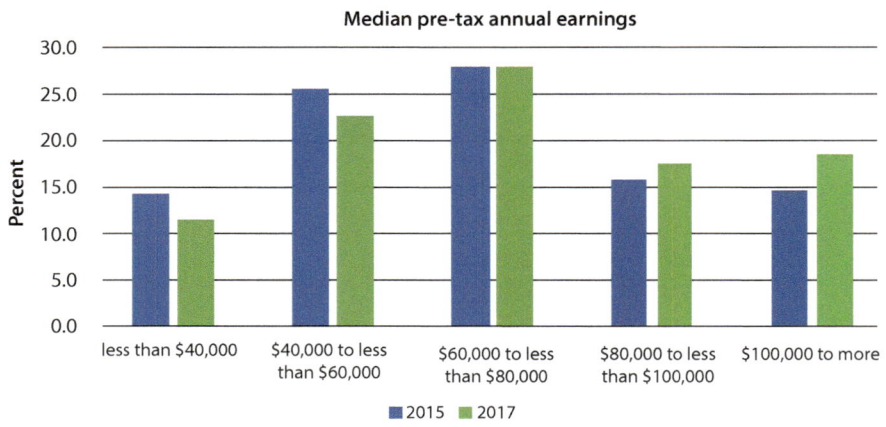

☒ **Fig. 4.6**   RN Median pre-tax annual earnings (National Councils for State Boards of Nursing 2020)

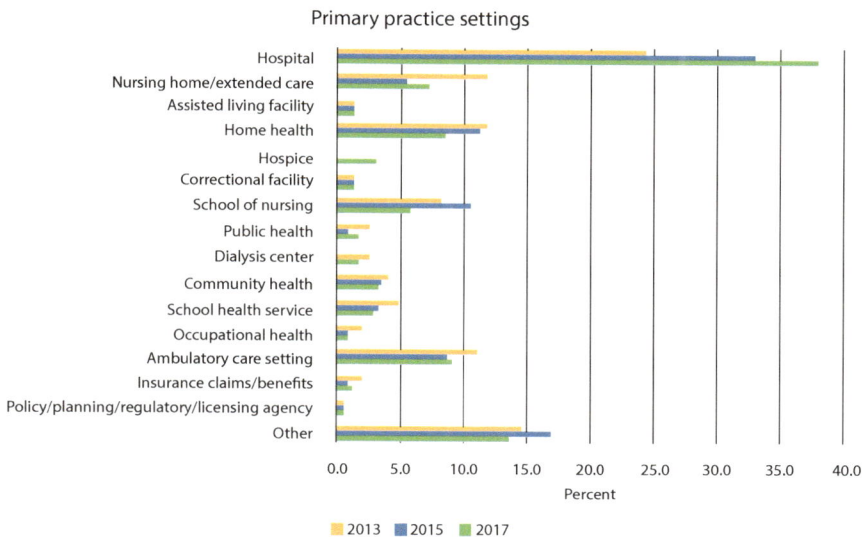

● **Fig. 4.7** Primary RN practice settings (National Councils for State Boards of Nursing 2020)

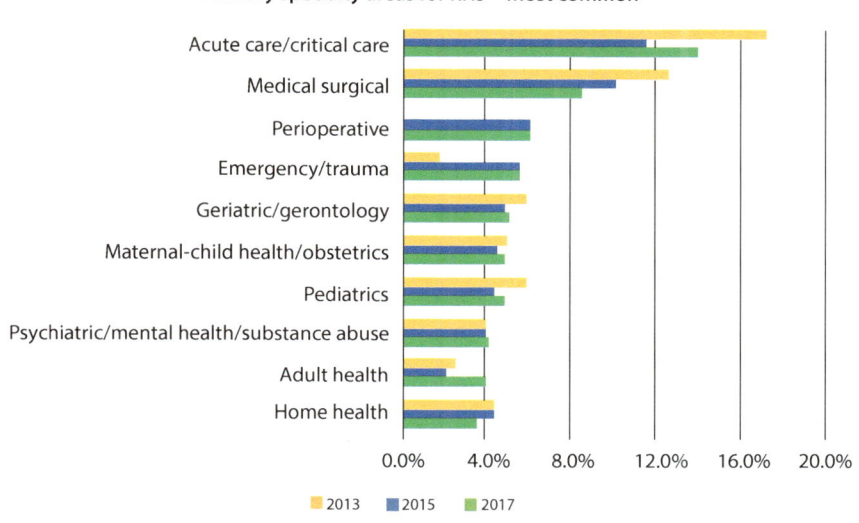

● **Fig. 4.8** Primary specialty area for RNs (National Councils for State Boards of Nursing 2020)

4.4.1 Diploma

These programs are limited in number and are based on clinical hours, which prepare you to take the NCLEX resulting in an RN license. Students can complete the program in 2 to 3 years. These programs were standard in the early

1900s and have progressively decreased in number, with only a handful still in existence in the United States. Nurses are trained in the hospital. Nurses do not receive a degree, and they receive a diploma certificate. This is important to consider as going back to school for a higher-level degree will be much more challenging in terms of time and money. The programs are relatively rare, and many are being phased out.

4

4.4.2 Associates Degree in Nursing (ADN)

A registered nurse (RN) can complete this program in 2 years and is eligible to take the NCLEX exam resulting in an RN license. Programs are typically offered in community college settings and trade schools.

4.4.3 Bachelor of Science in Nursing (BSN)

A registered nurse (RN) can earn a bachelor's degree through a traditional university and successfully pass the NCLEX resulting in an RN license. These programs take 4 years to complete. Accelerated programs are offered for those with a bachelor's degree in another field. Accelerated programs can take as little as 2 years to complete. For ADN prepared nurses, a interested in obtaining a BSN, time to complete a program is 1 to 2 years through online or hybrid programs. A hybrid program includes a combination of online and in-person classes and clinical.

4.4.3.1 Which One?—Diploma, ADN, or BSN?

For those deciding to seek the RN, options exist. The diploma, ADN, and BSN each lead to an RN license. The difference lies in the education behind the license, the opportunity for advancement, and, in some cases, salary. The American Association of Colleges of Registered nurses (RNs) (AACN) recognizes the BSN as the minimum education requirement for nursing professionals. While diploma programs do exist, it is not recommended as the educational needs are changing, and advancement beyond to another degree will require significant additional education. The BSN will cost more as the student takes extra course credit hours. The basic job duties do not differ, but BSN registered nurses (RNs) have more opportunities to take on additional responsibilities and move into more advanced positions. Some employers, especially Magnet recognized employers, prefer to hire BSN registered nurses (RNs). A Magnet Hospital is an honor awarded by the American Nurses Credentialing Center demonstrating excellence in nursing and patient care.

When choosing a nursing school, consider the following factors:

- Location: Is it close to where you live? Remember, you will be traveling to the school and surrounding hospitals as a student, and commute time may be a factor.

- Degree choice: Educate yourself in the various types of degrees. Decide which best meet your career goals for, both the long and short term.
- Accreditation: An accredited school has completed the accreditation process by a peer review board. Accreditation is important because it means the institution meets or exceeds minimum standards of quality.
- Size of the nursing school and class size: You may want to visit the school for a tour. Some students prefer smaller schools and others prefer larger schools. Larger school may have larger class sizes. There are pros and cons to both. Typically smaller schools offer more attention to students. Larger schools are often less expensive.
- Class schedules: When you visit the school, ask about the class schedule. Nursing school schedules typically include long days in the hospital in addition to classes and labs on campus.
- NCLEX exam pass rates: The NCLEX pass rate for graduates of the program is essential. Graduates want to complete their studies, pass NCLEX, obtain their RN license, and begin working. If the pass rate is low for a school, graduates are more likely to face the anxiety-provoking task of having to retake the NCELX and potentially losing an employment opportunity after graduation.

4.5 Master's Degree

There are several paths to get a master's degree. Some can enter a master's program after completion of the BSN. There are two types of MSN degrees. A non-APRN MSN is for those interested in a Clinical Nurse Leader (CNL) degree or Nurse Educator. The APRN is a degree for those interested in becoming an advanced practice registered nurse (RN). An APRN degree includes Nurse Practitioner (NP), Certified Nurse-Midwife (CNM), Clinical Nurse Specialist (CNS), or Certified Nurse Anesthetist (CRNA). After completing the program, the APRN must certified. Some APRNs require a doctorate, such as CRNAs. Other APRNs will likely follow in requiring the doctoral degree in the coming years. A master's degree can take 1–2 years to complete if the applicant has an ADN or BSN. Universities offer these programs. The delivery of education can be on campus or online. Costs vary with a minimum of $30,000 for a master's degree. The non-APRN masters registered nurse (RN) does not take a second licensure exam. APRNs do take a second licensure exam and have an expanded autonomy. In some states, APRNs can work independently and run their clinic and practice.

4.6 Doctor of Nursing Practice (DNP)

The DNP requires a minimum of 3 years of study and is offered through universities on campus or online. These programs prepare graduates for leadership positions in research, clinical care, patient outcomes, and system management. Courses aim to prepare graduates in advanced nursing care roles and fiscal

4

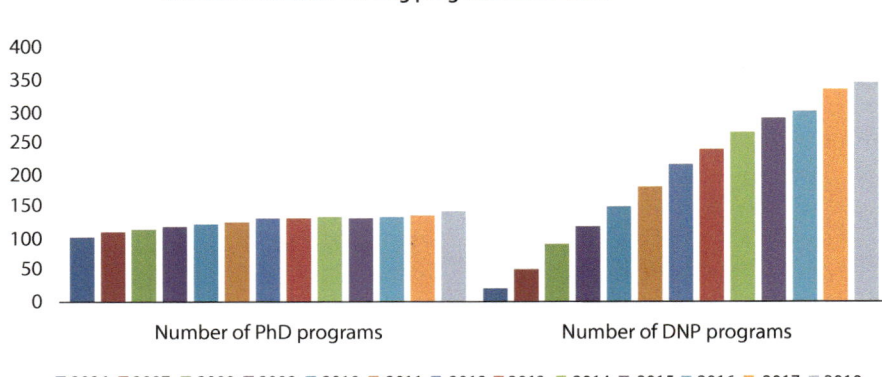

◘ Fig. 4.9   Growth in doctoral nursing programs (American Association of Colleges of Nursing 2020b)

responsibilities. While there is overlap between the two, the DNP is distinctive from a Masters degree. A DNP provides a foundation in evidence-based practice and improving patient outcomes. A DNP is a clinical doctorate and is the highest level of training in clinical nursing and a rapidly growing field as evidence by a significant increase in the number of programs across the US (◘ Fig. 4.9).

4.7 Advanced Practice Registered Nurses (APRNs)

An advanced practice registered nurse (RN) is a registered nurse (RN) who possesses advanced education and training. Nursing roles have evolved as healthcare delivery has changed. Many variations in nursing roles have developed.

4.7.1 APRN Credentialing or Certified Nurse? What Is the Difference?

Credentialing is a process used to designate a person who has met specific established standards set by a governmental or nongovernmental agent. This person is qualified to perform in a specialized area. A credential is a stamp of quality and achievement for employers and consumers. Through credentialing, others can know what to expect from a credentialed nurse. Credentials are typically renewed periodically to assure continued quality of the APRN. The largest number of credentialed APRNs are Nurse Practitioners (NP) (◘ Fig. 4.10).

A certification is a form of validating a person's educational and professional achievements. Certification is a formal process that recognizes and validates a per-

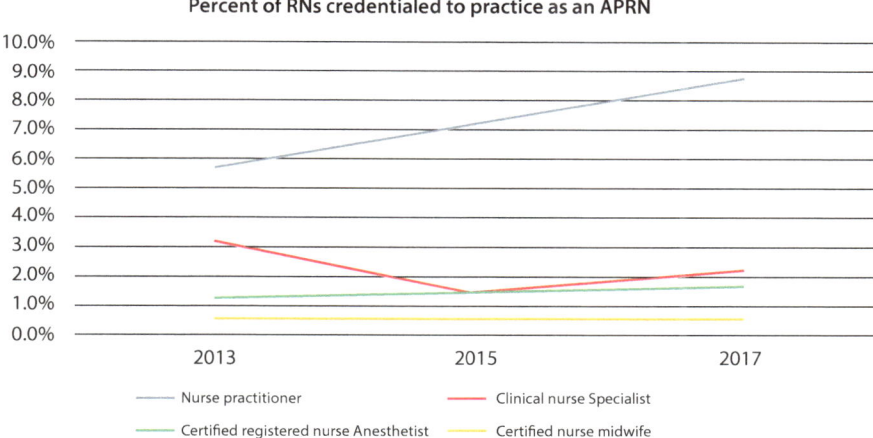

Fig. 4.10 RNs credentialed as APRNS (National Councils for State Boards of Nursing 2020)

son's qualifications in a specific specialty area. Certification is a process where a nongovernmental agency, organization, or association certifies a person licensed to practice in a specialized field. The person meets predetermined standards specified by the profession in their area of specialty practice.

Consensus Model for APRN Regulation

APRN specialties
Focus of practise beyond role and population focus linked to health care needs
Examples include but are not limited to: Oncology, Older Adults, Orthopedics, Nephrology, Palliative Care

Population FOCI

Licensure occurs at Levels of Role & Population Foci

| Family/ Individual across lifespan | Adult gerontology* | Neonatal | Pediatrics | Women's health/ gender-related | Psychiatric- mental health** |

APRN ROLES

| Nurse anesthetist | Nurse-midwife | Clinical Nurse specialist** | Nurse practitioner* |

American Nurses Credentialing Center (2020)

4

4.7.2 **APRN**

BSN prepared registered nurses (RNs) who meet criteria may pursue an advanced practice registered nurse (RN) (APRN) degree in several areas. The four recognized areas are certified nurse midwife (CNM), certified registered nurse anesthetist (CRNA) nurse practitioners (NP), and clinical nurse specialists (CNS). Each type of APRN plays a vital role in providing healthcare. APRNs practice with high levels of independence and responsibility across a wide variety of clinical settings APRNs treat and diagnose, manage chronic disease, and engage in continuous professional developments in their fields. An APRN must complete either a master's or doctoral program in their nursing specialty and must maintain licensing requirements as an RN. APRNs. are trained according to the consensus model which aligns APRN licensure, accreditation, certification and education. These areas represent the highest-paid branches of nursing. Each APRN plays a vital role in healthcare and the future of healthcare (Fig. 4.11).

APRNs:
- Treat and diagnose illness
- Advise the public on health issues
- Manage chronic disease
- Engage in continuous professional education (American Nurses Association 2020a)

 Fig. 4.11   Four types of APRNS

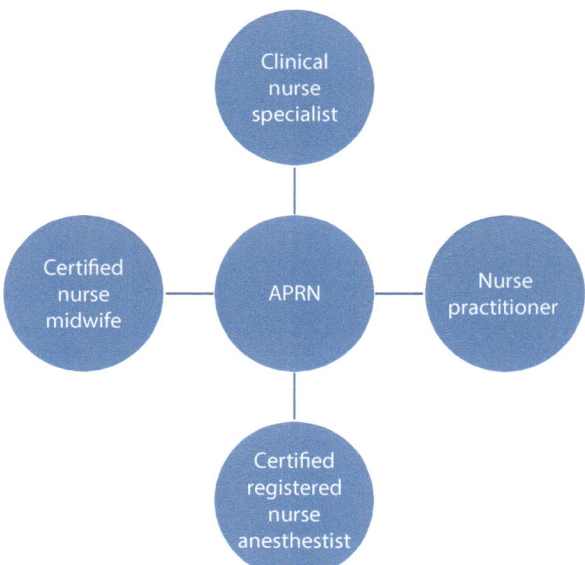

4.7.3 **Registered Nurse Practitioners (NP)**

According to the American Association of Nurse Practitioners (AANP), there are more than 270,000 NPs in the USA. In 2018, 68.7% of APRNs were nurse practitioners (◘ Fig. 4.12). Nurse practitioners provide primary, acute, and specialty healthcare services for patients across the lifespan. Nurse practitioners assess, diagnose, and treat illnesses and injuries. The majority of nurse practitioners (87%) are certified in an area of primary care. The mean salary of an NP is $105,903. Litigation against nurse practitioners is rare, with less than 1% being named as the primary defendant in a malpractice case. Their clinical focus areas range across the lifespan.

Nurse practitioners have been shown to ensure positive patient outcomes consistently. Unfortunately, there are many barriers to independent practice, and the scope of practice varies across state lines. Not all NPs practice independently, and nurse practitioners need to understand the range of training in the state where they practice (American Nurses Association 2020b; National Councils of State Boards of Nursing. 2019).

4.7.4 **NP Programs of Study**

Online and hybrid programs exist when seeking an NP program. A hybrid program is a mixture of face to face and online coursework. Students typically take 1 ½ to 3 years to complete their degree. Of course, the timeline varies based on whether the student is attending part-time or full-time. Programs offer master's or doctorate degrees. AACN encourages APRN students to obtain a DNP, a requirement has not been mandated, and master's programs are still available. A DNP will be mandated in the future. There are many nurse practitioner specialization areas (◘ Fig. 4.12).

◘ **Fig. 4.12** Total NP graduates 2008 to 2017 (Salsberg 2018)

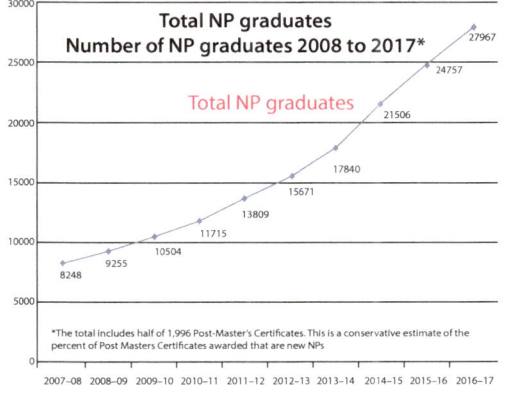

4

4.7.5 Types of NP

4.7.5.1 Neonatal Nurse Practitioner (NNP)

NNPs specialize in the care of acutely ill newborn infants who require postnatal care in neonatal intensive care units, emergency rooms, delivery rooms, or specialty clinics. NNPs have advanced skills in the psychosocial and physical assessment of newborns. They manage the transport of acutely ill babies when applicable across healthcare settings. The work environment is intense and fast paced. The NNP must be competent in technical equipment, ventilators, hemodynamic monitoring, assessment and care of acutely ill infants, central line management, skilled in working with families, and an interdisciplinary team player.

4.7.5.2 Acute Care Nurse Practitioner (ACNP)

ACNPs provide advanced care to acutely ill patients with complicated, critical, and chronic health conditions. ACNPs may work in emergency rooms, operating rooms, urgent care clinics, critical care units, or in a community-based environment. They may perform advanced invasive diagnostic and therapeutic procedures. They write prescriptions, interpret electrocardiogram (ECG) monitoring, assess patient responses to medications, and have other advanced skills used in the care of acutely ill patients. An ACNP can specialize in Gerontology and become an Adult-Gerontology Acute Care nurse Practitioner (AG-ACNP).

4.7.5.3 Certified Nurse-Midwife (CNM)

In 2018, 2.4% of APRNs were CNMs. As an APRN, CNMs have higher salary opportunities because of their advanced skills and responsibilities. The median full-time earnings were $102,115. A CNM provides specialized care in women's reproductive healthcare and childbirth. They attend births, perform annual exams, give counseling, and write prescriptions. CNMs offer family planning services, prenatal care, and education for parents. They collaborate with healthcare professionals and provide training programs specific to reproductive health and care. They provide education on sexual health, menopause, and treat gynecological disorders. CNMs can work with a group of providers or start their own practice depending on the scope of practice in their state.

4.7.5.4 Clinical Registered Nurse (RN) Specialists (CNSs)

Clinical nurse specialists have been part of healthcare since the 1960s. Over time CNSs have become widely accepted as advanced practice registered nurses (RNs) who impact healthcare by providing efficient and effective healthcare services. In 2018, 19% of APRNs were CNSs. The median full-time earnings were $95,723. CNSs practice in a framework known as the three spheres of influence: patient, nurse and system. CNSs diagnose, treat, and manage patients. CNSs provide expertise and support to registered nurse (RN) caring for patients. They help drive practice change throughout the organization and ensure evidence-based care, and best practices are upheld to ensure ideal patient outcomes.

CNSs are expert clinicians with advanced education and clinical training in a variety of healthcare settings. Their specialty can be defined in a variety of ways.

- Population: such as pediatric, geriatric, and women's health
- Settings: such as critical care and psychiatric
- Disease: such as diabetes or oncology
- Type of care: such as rehabilitation or emergency care
- Type of health problem: such as wound, pain, orthopedic

CNS practice varies from state to state. Each state's licensing board regulates the scope of practice for CNSs. Most states require advanced certification. For example, certification exams include adult/gerontology, pediatrics, and neonatal (National Association for Clinical Nurse Specialists 2020).

4.7.5.5 Certified Registered Nurse (RN) Anesthetists (CRNAs)

In 2018, 9.3% of APRNs were CRNAs. While the general RN workforce is 9% male, 41% of CRNAs are male. The median full-time earnings were $161,000. CRNAs work in collaboration with surgeons, anesthesiologists, dentists, podiatrists, and other professionals to manage the safe administration of anesthesia to patients. CRNAs provide a full range of anesthesia and pain management services to patients. They monitor patients while they receive anesthesia and after recovery from anesthesia. They provide care during simple and complex procedures (▶ https://www.nursingworld.org/practice-policy/workforce/what-is-nursing/aprn/, ▶ https://www.nursingjobs.com/five-tips-for-advancing-your-nursing-career/).

4.8 Research-Focused Doctorate: Ph.D.

Ph.D. programs prepare registered nurse (RN) scholars and researchers with theoretical knowledge in nursing healthcare delivery. Ph.D. programs take 3 to 5 years to complete and are offered through universities. Registered nurses (RNs) with Ph.D. play a role in leading the healthcare system and the implementation of policies that can change the direction of nursing and hospitals at all levels. The Ph.D. is considered a terminal degree, the highest degree and RN can obtain. Registered nurses (RNs) with a Ph.D. teach, conduct research, evaluate programs, write and lead healthcare organizations. The sky is the limit with this type of degree. Typically Ph.D. registered nurses (RNs) are found in a variety of practice settings. No matter where they work, they are commonly expected to conduct research as one of their job duties.

4.8.1 Which Doctoral Degree? DNP or Ph.D.?

4

Both the Ph.D. and DNP are considered terminal degrees for nurses. Both a nurse is a clinical expert in his or her field of study. There are differences between the two degrees (◘ Table 4.1). A Ph.D. is a research-focused degree, and a DNP is a clinical practice-focused degree. The degree path should be chosen based on the nurses career goals. If a nurse is aiming to expand knowledge in a practice field such as nurse practitioner or CRNA, a DNP path should be chosen. If a nurse is hoping to move into research, leadership, and academia a Ph.D. should be selected. Ph.D. prepared nurses conduct research and use research to improve patient care and advance the science of the nursing profession. The curriculum is research-based, and original research is required to complete a dissertation. They may also teach nursing students. There are no patient care clinical hours in the curriculum. (◘ Table 4.2)

◘ Table 4.1 DNP and Ph.D. comparison

	Doctor of Nursing Practice	**Doctor of Philosophy**
Program of Study	Aims to prepare nurses at the highest levels of clinical practice Competencies are described in AACN essentials of DNP	Aims to develop nurse researchers Educated in theory research methodology Emphasizes the role of researcher and faculty role
Faculty	Doctorate with expertise in the specific teaching area Senior leader Clinical leaders Advanced of knowledge in the practice area	Research doctorate in a related field Senior-level research funding Program of research consistent with are of the program focus Research methodology expertise
Students	Committed to a career in practice and or service leadership Orientated towards improving care outcomes	Dedicated to a research career Orientated towards developing new knowledge and establishment of a research program in a discipline
Resources	Mentors in leadership positions across various healthcare settings which may or may not be in nursing State of the science resources Access to diverse practice settings Access to databases in practice settings and evaluation data	Mentors in research and advanced practice role preparation Active programs of research Access to dissertation support dollars Support for the state of science information, communication, and management
Program Outcome	Contributes to the advancement of healthcare via direct service or policy change Program accredited in specialized accreditation field	Development of new knowledge, research contribution, scholarly products that advance nursing science

◘ **Table 4.2** Comparison of registered nurse (RN) career levels

Level	Typical Education Requirement	Current number in US	Mean salary in US	Scope of practice
CNA	75-hour vocational course	1.5 million	$24,000 ($22/ hour)	Limited range of procedures (vital signs, dispensing medications, bathing patients, transferring patients). Work under the supervision of RNs
LPN	1-year vocation course	700,000	$41,000	Administers injections, therapeutic massage, prepares patients for surgical procedures, maintains patient records, changes dressings, some intravenous medication management. Communicate patient needs to medical staff
RN	Associate of Science in Nursing or Bachelor of Science in Nursing	2.7 million	$71,000 ($34/ hour)	Make a nursing diagnosis, supervise CNAs and LPNs, administer and monitor medications (including intravenous), perform and lead emergency response (BLS, ACLS, PALS), wound care, adminster chemotherapy, adminster blood products, develop a plan of care, assess patient, accept provider verbal orders, admit and discharge patients, lead and supervise RNs
APRN	Masters or Doctorate	$150,000	$113,000 ($54/ hour)	CNM, NP, CRNA, CNS
Advanced Practice Nursing	Masters or Doctorate			Registered nurse (RN) researchers, registered nurse (RN) educators, registered nurse (RN) leaders

Navigating the options for nursing education can be daunting. The key is to explore your goals and how they align with your unique career goals which align with your values, beliefs, and skills.

4

Strategies

Strategy 1. Buzzfeed.com offers a quiz to determine if you are ready to go back to school. ▶ https://www.buzzfeed.com/aberardelli31/this-quiz-will-tell-you-if-youre-ready-for-school-hfiw9v3cr

Strategy 2. US News and World Report offer a quiz to determine if you are prepared to plunge into graduate school. ▶ https://www.usnews.com/education/best-graduate-schools/articles/2016/06/07/quiz-are-you-ready-to-take-the-grad-school-plunge

❓ Activity

1. Create a table that aligns your goals from ▶ Chap. 2 with ▶ Chaps. 3 and 4 career path development. Use the SMART goal acronym to develop your goals. Evaluate if your short-term goals align with long-term goal achievement.

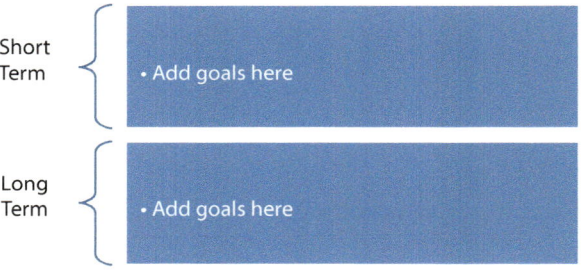

2. Conduct an environmental scan of what is out there. Explore what interests you, what is the requirement to achieve what interests you, and develop a path to get there.
3. Ask a registered nurse (RN) if you can buy them coffee and ask them the following questions.

    (a) How did you get where you are today?
    (b) What do you love most about your job?
    (c) What do you dislike about your job?
    (d) What was your most difficult challenge in achieving your goals?
    (e) What are your most significant rewards?

Use their responses to guide you in your decision-making.

4. Quizony.com offers a quiz to help you determine what kind of nurse you should be. ▶ https://www.quizony.com/what-kind-of-registered nurse (RN)-should-i-be/index.html

Vignettes

Vignette 1

How did you get through your doctoral program while working and managing a busy home life?

I am not entirely sure when I look back at that time. I do know I was determined and used every free moment I had to work on my assignments. Once I got a routine going, I found out there were lots of opportunities to complete my school work. Don't underestimate the value of getting organized; when you organize your assignments, you don't waste time finding information.

How did you pay for all the expenses?

I used my resources and took the time to talk with others and find out where small scholarships could be applied for, every little bit helped.

How did you decide on what program to study?

I thought to myself, what would I like to do for the rest of my career? I did not know about salary. I just thought about what I was interested in. I am happy I used this approach; I am now comfortable in my chosen path and make enough money too.

Vignette 2

What do you like about being a nurse researcher? What don't you like?

I've been a research nurse for 7 months now. It's the specialty I got into right after graduation. I was able to find work in this area because I had worked in research for 3 years before I went to nursing school. Just like any job, there are things I like and things I dislike, so I will just make a little list.

Things I love about being a research nurse:

1. Getting paid to read new study protocols and learn about new drugs, devices, diseases, and treatments. I have always loved school and learning, so this suits me. I think it helps that I especially love pharmacology, but this is not necessary to enjoy the job.

2. Educating patients about the study and the new drug/device and talking with them about their participation. Not everyone should be part of a clinical trial, so the informed consent discussion is critical. Some studies enroll healthy volunteers who will be asked to take the drug so that its safety/tolerability can be established, and some studies are enrolling people diagnosed with diseases that might be treated by the new drug (e.g., cancer and cancer treatments). Other studies are designed purely to answer a practical or theoretical question about the drug (e.g., does it have an effect on lab values?). The purpose of the trial makes a big difference for the patient, and I work hard to make sure they understand the point and the risks/benefits of the study. I see this as my primary nursing duty when I'm on the job.

3. Caring for my patients! If I have drawn some labs for the study, and I see some abnormalities in the results, I have to take care of that. I consult with my proviers and inform the patient, making referrals as needed. This is my favorite part of my job.

4

4. Highly regular hours, almost no weekends or evenings. 8 am-4 pm M-F with very occasional exceptions dictated by certain studies (some studies might require weekend dosing, etc.)
5. The physicians are generally very respectful of us—they know that we know a study inside and out, and they take our opinion seriously.

Things I don't like about being a research nurse:
1. Depending on the particular job, patient contact may or may not be a considerable part of the day. Some places you will work only with charts/data/paperwork, and others you will spend maybe half the day with patients.
2. There is always a lot of paperwork in nursing, but research takes it to a whole new level. HUGE amounts of paperwork related to the FDA, the sponsor, the patient chart, the institutional review board, the facility...There is always the anxiety that you've missed something or haven't reported something.

Vignette 3
Interview with Pam Cipriano, past president of ANA. In this interview, Dr. Cipriano talks about how she became a nurse, the value of nursing, and how she is working to give nursing a voice in healthcare (Thew 2018).

References

American Association of Colleges of Nursing (2020a) Nursing fact sheet. Retrieved from: https://www.aacnnursing.org/News-Information/Fact-Sheets/Nursing-Fact-Sheet

American Association of Colleges of Nursing (2020b) DNP fact sheet. Retrieved from: https://www.aacnnursing.org/News-Information/Fact-Sheets/DNP-Fact-Sheet

American Nurses Association (2020a) Advanced practice registered nurse. What is APRN nursing? Retrieved from: https://www.nursingworld.org/practice-policy/workforce/what-is-nursing/aprn/

American Nurses Association (2020b) Advanced practice registered nurse. NP fact sheet Retrieved from https://www.aanp.org/about/all-about-nps/np-fact-sheet

American Nurses Credentialing Center (2020) Consensus model for APRN regulation. https://www.apna.org/m/pages.cfm?pageid=3745

Fitzpatrick (2017) 301 careers in nursing. Springer

National Association for Clinical Nurse Specialists. (2020) What is CNS? Retrieved from: https://nacns.org/about-us/what-is-a-cns/

National Councils for State Boards of Nursing (2020) National nursing workforce study. Retrieved from: https://www.ncsbn.org/workforce.htm

National Councils of State Boards of Nursing. (2019) NCSBN publishes findings from survey of advanced practice registered nurses with collaborative practice agreements. Retrieved from: https://www.ncsbn.org/13374.htm

Salsberg (2018) Changes in the pipeline of new NPs and RNs: Implications for Health Care Delivery and Educational Capacity. Health Affairs. Retrieved from: https://www.healthaffairs.org/do/10.1377/hblog20180524.993081/full/

Thew (2018) The interview: American nurses association President Pamela Cipriano. Health Leaders. Retrieved from: https://www.healthleadersmedia.com/nursing/interview-american-nurses-association-president-pamela-f-cipriano

Strategic Path Development

Contents

Charting YOUR Career Path: Internal Strategies

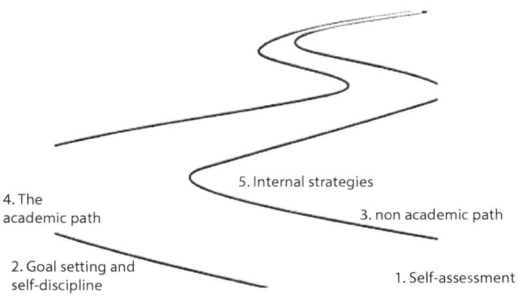

Contents

© Springer Nature Switzerland AG 2020
J. M. Manning, *The Path to Building a Successful Nursing Career*,
https://doi.org/10.1007/978-3-030-50023-8_5

You will never feel truly satisfied by work until you are satisfied by life.
—*Heather Schuck*

You may not realize it when it happens, but a kick in the teeth may be the best thing in the world for you. — *Walt Disney*

5.1 Introduction

Taking on an activity for its own sake without a visible reward, may stem from feelings such as happiness, anger or sadness, thoughts such as (I must finish my work by the deadline), values, and goals. Motivation is the reason for peoples actions and willingness often stemming from wants or desires. Motivation can originate from intrinsic or extrinsic sources. Internal motivation is enjoyable and exciting. Internal motivation is behavior driven by internal rewards within the individual which are naturally satisfying. External motivation requires earning of external awards or avoiding punishment. For example, one may read a book because it is interesting. Each one of us is motivated differently, and while one sees a task as intrinsically motivating, another may see the extrinsic motivation.

The concepts described in this chapter include internal motivation, risk-taking, and work–life balance. Risk taking is the decision to take a risk and acting on the decision. Work life balance is the balance between work activities and personal life activities.

5.2 Internal Motivation

Internal motivation is a behavior that is driven by internal rewards and arises from inside the individual. It is like solving a puzzle for the purpose of solving it, not because you have to. Motivation engages one in behavior that occurs from within a person because it satisfies them. The person undertakes the activity for its own sake, without an external reward. Internal motivation, because of the internal drive, is often easy to maintain concentration, and a person will do it regardless of the reward because the motivation comes from inside them. Internal motivation can be subject to moods. When you are feeling down, internal motivation can be negatively impacted.

When describing motivation, specifically internal motivation, it is essential to acknowledge external motivation as well. External motivation affects motivation; it comes from outside the individual. It is motivated by solving a problem for a reward, such as money or recognition from others. External motivation is easy to manufacture through the use of a reward system. Consider household chores in children, such as taking out the garbage. Most are not internally motivated to do household chores. But the use of a reward system such as an allowance helps motivate one to do the task. The reward makes the chore bearable. Unfortunately, because the task is not internally motivated, procrastination often results.

Unfortunately, internal motivation does not support everything we do, and many accept a challenge because of internally motivating reasons.

If you fear failure, you may not activate the goal initially. To fix this fear, remember to look at all of the possible outcomes and worst-case scenarios. Ask yourself if you fail, will it be the worst possible thing to happen? Consider the consequences of not activating the goal and the adverse outcomes associated with it. Consider using this potentially harmful outcome to jumpstart you into activating your goal.

Moving beyond the internally motivating goal and into some of the new goals which require perseverance, requires some external motivation. Acknowledgment of the goal and why you embarked upon it and the use of rewards along the way can help you persevere through a long-term goal you set out to achieve. Consider what you need to do, not the time it will take to complete the task. This approach helps time pass and ensures you focus on the activities necessary to achieve the goal. Use a tracking system to monitor your progress with small goals built into it. The tracking system helps you focus on how much you have done and how much left to do. If you begin to just not feel like working on your goal, start with getting organized. Being able to move right into working on a goal can help you get to work faster and procrastinate less. If you become apathetic or delay a task, you need to get motivated by eliminating excuses, remember why you activated this goal, building in rewards, and persevere!

Factors which promote intrinsic motivation include:

- *Curiosity*

Curiosity pushes us to explore and learn for learning and mastering. We learn more efficiently when we are exploring something we are interested in learning more about. Motivation follows curiosity.

- *Challenge*

A challenge helps us work at an optimal level and work toward a goal. Many successful people are inspired by the challenges they face and turn a problem or challenge as a source of motivation.

- *Control*

Control sources from an intrinsic desire to control change and make decisions to influence an outcome. Control is a cognitive strategy that aims to strengthen motivation.

- *Recognition*

Recognition is the innate need to be appreciated and recognized by others. Many people respond to appreciation and recognition because it confirms the value of their work. Motivation follows recognition.

- Cooperation

Cooperation is the feeling of personal satisfaction when we help others and work together on a shared goal. It satisfies our need for belonging.

5

- **Competition**

Competition increases the importance we place on doing well and poses a personal challenge. Some are motivated by competition because it allows them to satisfy the need to win and a reason to improve performance.

- **Fantasy**

Fantasy is the use of positive mental images to stimulate behavior. This links cognition to motivation and behavior, which puts a person into action.

Case Example 5.1 Examples of Internal Motivation

Internal Motivation Examples:
- volunteering because you feel content and fulfilled rather than needing it to meet a school or work requirement
- going for a run because you find it relaxing or are trying to beat a personal record, not to win a competition
- taking on more responsibility at work because you enjoy being challenged and feeling accomplished, rather than to get a raise or promotion
- painting a picture because you feel calm and happy when you paint rather than selling your art to make money
- participating in a sport because it's fun and you enjoy it rather than doing it to win an award
- learning a new language because you like experiencing new things, not because your job requires it
- spending time with someone because you enjoy their company and not because they can further your social standing
- cleaning because you prefer a tidy space rather than doing it to avoid making your spouse angry
- playing cards because you enjoy the challenge instead of playing to win money
- exercising because you enjoy physically challenging your body instead of doing it to lose weight or fit into an outfit

---

Case Example 5.2 Strategies to Improve Intrinsic Motivation

Intrinsic Motivation Strategies
- Help someone in need, whether it's a friend who could use a hand at home or lending a hand at a soup kitchen.
- Create a list of things you genuinely love to do or have always wanted to do and choose something on the list to do whenever you have time or are feeling uninspired.
- Participate in the competition and focus on the camaraderie and how well you perform instead of on winning.

- Before starting a task, visualize a time that you felt proud and accomplished and focus on those feelings as you work to conquer the task.
- Look for the fun in work and other activities or find ways to make tasks engaging for yourself.
- Find meaning by focusing on your value, the purpose of a task, and how it helps others.
- Keep challenging yourself by setting attainable goals that focus on mastering a skill, not on external gains.

Internal motivation can be used in all life aspects. The development of internal motivation can be an effective way to improve performance. Simple steps like altering the focus of internal rewards such as satisfaction and enjoyment can better help you motivate yourself and others.

» Being told you are appreciated is one of the simplest, yet most incredible things you can hear. —author unknown

There are many ways to improve internal motivation. Consider the following:
- Look for fun at work.
- Identify ways to make tasks more engaging.
- Find meaning through a value focus and the purpose of the task as well as how it helps others.
- Challenge yourself by setting goals that are attainable and master a skill.
- Help others in need.
- Increase your awareness of what you love by creating a list of what you have always wanted to do. Work towards something on the list.
- Participate in healthy competition and performance.
- Visualize what makes you proud and accomplished. Use this visual image to focus on those feelings.

Through these strategies, one can improve motivation, clarify purpose, and ultimately improve performance. Changing your focus to that of satisfaction and enjoyment can motivate you and others (Legg 2019; Wolfe 2020; Robbins 2007).

5.3 Risk-Taking

Jeff Bezos quit a well-paying job as a senior vice-president working in a hedge fund to start up his company, which we all know as Amazon in his garage. He took a significant risk when making this career change. Career decisions are a risk. If you are aiming to build your nursing career, you are already considering a change. How will you know if you should take a risk or stay on the current and potentially "safer" option? Hopefully, you have already realized that this risk will not come

5

easy. There will be blood, sweat, and tears involved. Additionally, there will need to be hard work, self-reflection, and uncertainness and, ultimately, risk-taking.

In a book by Wendy Sachs titled, *Fearless and Free*, the author describes how smart women pivot and relaunch their careers. The author begins by stating, success and achievement is not handed to us and doesn't land in our lap. She goes on to say one should start with small goals to begin the momentum. Rejection is also mentioned, which is a natural occurrence with any risk. You may not hear back from those you contact. The key is to move on to the next strategy and remain persistent. Don't give up! Once a comfort level is achieved with small goals, the more significant risk may not be as intimidating.

Life is full of risk, and every decision we make involves a level of risk. Some changes are apparent, others are less overt. For example, when you woke up today, you decided to get out of bed and possibly have breakfast. You may have decided to feed your children or pet (if you have any). When you drove to work, you decided to stop at a stop sign (or roll through it), depending on how you handled each of these decisions involved some level of risk.

The study of risk and risk-taking dates back to 3200 BC where deciding to take a chance was contemplated. Today, risk is defined in a variety of ways, like determining the risk of losing money in a company or the threat of starting a business or the risk of staying safe. Risk is a subjective concept, and not everyone similarly will agree upon the level of risk in specific situations.

When describing risk, it is essential to acknowledge individuals and groups. An individual evaluates their own risk based on their knowledge in the situation and evaluation of the risk factors. In group settings, group polarization or group think comes into play. People take more risks when they are in groups. An average decision can become a significant belief when a group of people holds the same idea. There are many examples in our history where group think was deadly, Chernobyl, Space Shuttle Challenger, and Pearl Harbor. One should be cautious to avoid group polarizing as it can have a positive or negative impact on you depending on how you decide in proceeding or not proceeding in a risk situation.

5.4   Maslow's Hierarchy of Needs

In 1970, Maslow published a Hierarchy of Needs. The levels build upon each other and include physiological, safety, love/belonging, esteem, and self-actualization (◘ Fig. 5.1). Physiological needs include basic needs such as air, food, water, warmth, and sleep. These are basic needs for sustaining and creating life. The next level is safety and consists of security, stability, authority, protection, freedom from fear, and shelter. The third level is love/belonging and includes psychological needs such as belongingness and love. The fourth level comprises self-esteem, confidence, achievement, respect of others, and by others. The top level is achieved after satisfying all of the other levels and the self begins to emerge through self-fulfillment. People can view that they have to give or contribute to others at this level. They desire self-fulfillment. Not everyone achieves this level.

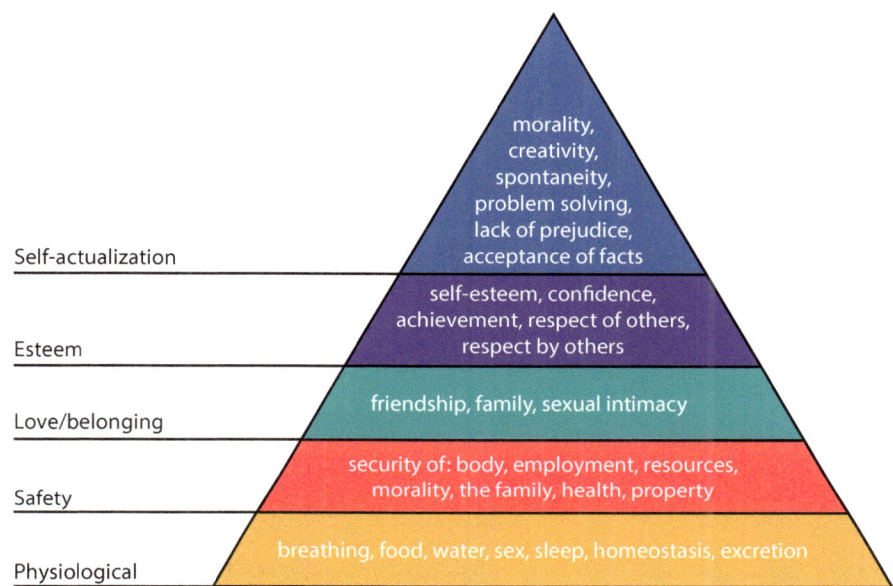

Self-actualization — morality, creativity, spontaneity, problem solving, lack of prejudice, acceptance of facts

Esteem — self-esteem, confidence, achievement, respect of others, respect by others

Love/belonging — friendship, family, sexual intimacy

Safety — security of: body, employment, resources, morality, the family, health, property

Physiological — breathing, food, water, sex, sleep, homeostasis, excretion

◻ **Fig. 5.1** Maslow's hierarchy of needs

Through risk-taking, more opportunities become available. There are some essential tips to avoid when considering risk-taking.

- Don't quit your job hastily due to a bad day or week.
- Don't participate in illegal or unethical activities.
- Don't take a pay cut that you cannot afford.
- Don't overstep your boundaries. For example, don't speak for your organization when you do not have the authority. Do not undermine your boss's authority. Respect for your organization and your boss is not a risk you want to violate.
- Lastly, do not take a risk into the complete unknown. Gather information and evaluate risk versus benefit.

There are several risks you should consider. First, "ask for more." If you want more challenges in your job, ask for more challenges. You should always be networking above your pay grade and exploring opportunities that increase your skill level and challenge you. Next, do not think of salary as your goal. For some, this may seem counterintuitive as they measure their success based on their payroll. You need to consider the big picture. The salary is one part. There are other vital components, such as non-monetary perks and benefits. Sonja Lyubomirsky, a positive psychology researcher, describes happiness as a deep sense of meaning and purpose. You will not achieve satisfaction by solely choosing a career based on salary.

5

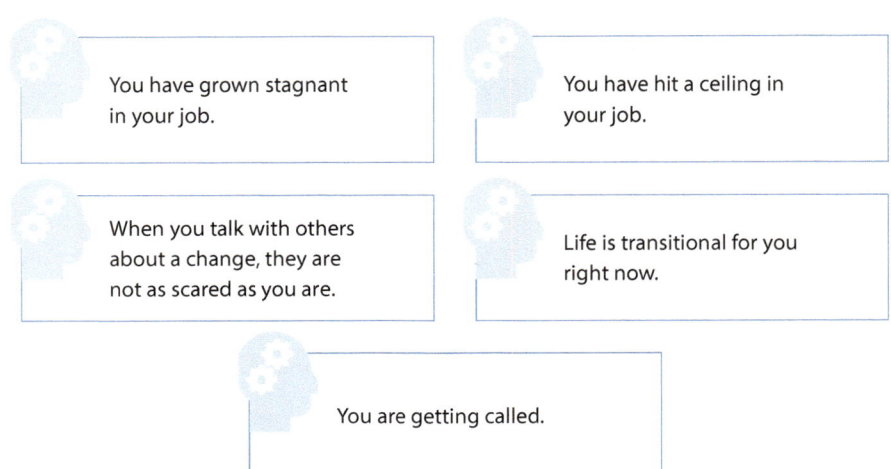

You have grown stagnant in your job.

You have hit a ceiling in your job.

When you talk with others about a change, they are not as scared as you are.

Life is transitional for you right now.

You are getting called.

◼ **Fig. 5.2** Signs you are ready to take a risk

Some signs you are prepared to take are risk include (◼ Fig. 5.2):

— You have grown stagnant in your job. Boredom is destructive in your professional and personal life. When you are bored, you do not give 100% effort. Details become less critical. You are less thoughtful and uninspired. If you have grown stagnant in your job, you may be ready for a new career path.

— You have hit the ceiling in your job. While your work life can be enjoyable and rewarding while not actively being promoted, it is critical to evaluate if you are limiting your potential. If you hit the ceiling in your job, and something is telling you to do more, don't ignore that feeling. If you do, you may become unengaged and resentful. Your instincts are a good indicator you are seeking a risk or new opportunity. Build a support system and develop a large safety net if you are unsure about taking the risk.

— When you talk with others about a change, they are not as scared as you are. Some people spend exurbanite time evaluating a change and fear the change. When discussing with a trusted colleague or friend, they are surprised the friend is not alarmed. You may need to re-evaluate if your concerns are overblown and weigh the reward compared to the risk being considered. Be sure to discuss your risk with two to three people you trust. Use their input to help make your best decision to take a chance.

— Life is transitional for you right now. During transitional phases of life, self-concepts change. There is a natural desire to reconfigure work life. Transitions include major relocations, beginning or ending a life partnership, empty nesting, losing a loved one, recovering from a health challenge, or realizing you can retire. If you are in transition, you may feel the need to re-evaluate your career path. This may be the push you need to move closer to what you want in life.

— You are getting called. A calling to a new project or career change may be the push you need for a change. Knowing you can make money while pursuing a calling is confusing. Many people question the motive to pursue a life calling. Those who align careers with callings have a significant impact on the world. You should explore this calling as it may be a more significant risk not to.

5.5 Work–Life Balance

Work–life balance is a common buzz word and an essential aspect of a healthy work environment. When one maintains a healthy balance between work and personal life, there is a reduction in stress and workplace burnout. When one is chronically stressed, the consequences can physically manifest in the form of hypertension, digestive troubles, chronic aches and pains, and cardiovascular problems. Mental health can also be impacted in the way of depression, anxiety, and insomnia. Long work hours can lead to burnout exhibited by fatigue, mood swings, irritability, and reduction in work performance.

Work–life balance is unique to the individual and varies across generational groups. It is essential to work where the culture is healthy. Employees should be happy in their jobs, and they come to work for more than a paycheck. Working conditions should offer opportunities for professional growth and social connections. Leaders in the workplace should be aware of the work environment and strive to maximize productivity.

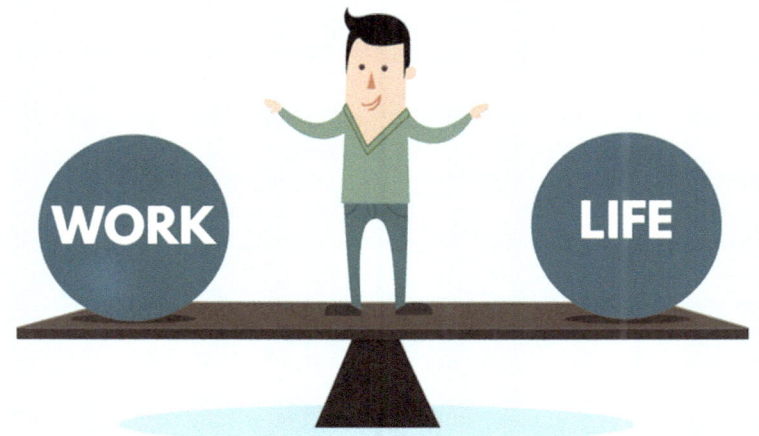

There are many strategies which guide ways to improve your work–life balance:

- Donate your time, expertise, or finances to something you believe in and stand for.
- Find a mentor to provide advice and insight. A mentor can be formal or informal. Ongoing meetings should occur with open dialogue and feedback.
- Plan vacation days and days off in advance. Each year 768 million vacation days go unused, and this number is increasing each year. It is essential to take your time off. If a vacation is not in your budget, a staycation is an important option. One should not feel guilty about taking time off. Productivity increases when workers use their vacation time each year (Jacobsen 2015; Kohll 2018; McCarthy 2018).
- Prioritize critical high priority tasks and do them first.
  - Differentiate nonnegotiables from other functions that are not important.
- Take time to rest mentally and physically.
  - It is essential to get adequate sleep each night, 8 hours is essential.
  - Ensure you have a strategy to recharge daily. For example, completing a gratitude journal, mindfulness, thank someone who you appreciate. Also, ensure you take time to transition between work and home to help you unwind. You can recharge with brief strategies, as little as 15 minutes.
- Add exercise as part of your daily routine. Daily exercise is essential and should amount to 150 minutes of moderate aerobic activity or 75 minutes of vigorous aerobic activity each week (Laskowski 2020).
- Declutter
  - Visual clutter makes you less productive and increases stress. Decluttering is a daily process. Focus on everyday tasks such as washing clothes and dishes at least every other day. From there, ensure you are not contributing to your clutter by putting your put things away as you use them. If items do not have a place to go, ensure you prioritize creating a place where they go. There are lots of books on minimalist lifestyles. If you have too much "stuff," you may want to read some of the books to find ways to minimize the clutter in your life. Some suggestions:
    - Minimalism: Live a Meaningful Life by Joshua Fields Millburn
    - The Joy of Less, A Minimalist Living Guide: How to Declutter, Organize and Simplify Your Life by Francine Jay
- Scheduling
  - Identify your most productive time frame and use that time for productivity. You can identify your most productive time by keeping a journal of how you spend your time and noting patterns of inactivity. Note when you have high energy work time. The key is to find what time of day you can focus the best. For most of us, late morning or around noon is our most productive time. Track your progress and adjust as you discover your most productive time.
- Organize your life
  - Organization begins with a calendar. You can use online or paper calendars. Calendars help you plan time to prepare for upcoming events. They help you track deadlines. They can help keep you informed. A calendar eases anxiety as you do not have to check on dates, times, and locations continually. Everything is in one place. A calendar helps you to know when you are available; you avoid double booking or over-committing. Use a tool that works for you, such as a paper calendar, or online calendar.

Strategies

Complete these free online quizzes:

Strategy 1. Complete the risk-taking test on psychtests.com ▶ https://testyourself. psychtests.com/testid/2122

Strategy 2. Complete the work–life balance quiz on business news daily.

do I have a healthy work-life balance?

▶ https://www.businessnewsdaily.com/8108-work-life-balance-quiz.html

❓ Activity

Answer the following questions to determine if you're work-life is imbalanced:

1. Are you out of shape? Try to make extra time for exercise. Even 20 minutes per day can improve your health and mood. Choose activities that work for you, either alone or with others. Plan for work meals to avoid fast food options.
2. Do you miss events due to an overbooked schedule? When friends call, do you have time to talk? Do you miss your child's events? Do you have to give up the activities you planned because you don't have time. A strategy to improve this issue is to say no to the right people. Aim to streamline routine tasks such as auto payments to manage bills. Create to-do lists and revise daily as tasks are completed. Use an online calendar for planning everything (work and home life).
3. Do you obsess over small details to the point it interferes with work life? If you are more than a perfectionist and struggle with anxiety or OCD? You may want to consider mindfulness techniques or other types of treatments to minimize anxiety.
4. Do you have a cluttered workspace? Clutter combined with long hours can cause stress and burnout. Try the TRAFing method. T = trash, R = refer, A = act, or F = file. This process can help you keep your space clean. Regularly clean and ensure you set boundaries for when the mess gets out of control.
5. Do you always work overtime? Staying late or coming in early to impress others can become a negative strategy in regard to home life and increase the risk for burnout. Working 60 hours weeks does not equate to being a good employee. Instead, focus on boundary setting. During work, focus on work. At home, focus on home. Ensure you have social groups outside of work to ensure you take a break from work. Also, develop nonwork-related hobbies.
6. Is your social life imbalanced? Do you sacrifice family time over work time? Social time is critical for balance. Ensure you schedule social events on your calendar, so you don't overbook.
7. Do you have a short fuse and a temper? You may need to explore strategies to manage anger and reflective strategies to explore why your temper is poor.
8. Do you get adequate sleep? Do work concerns keep you up at night? Poor sleep habits are a reliable indicator of poor work–life balance. Aim to create sleep routines.
9. What is your best time of day? Complete this quiz: ▶ https://www.gotoquiz. com/what_s_your_best_time_of_day
10. Complete this worksheet. How balanced is your current work/life vs. your preferred? If you are imbalanced, begin strategies on how you can realign your work–life balance. (◻ Fig. 5.3)

□ Fig. 5.3   Work–life balance
worksheet

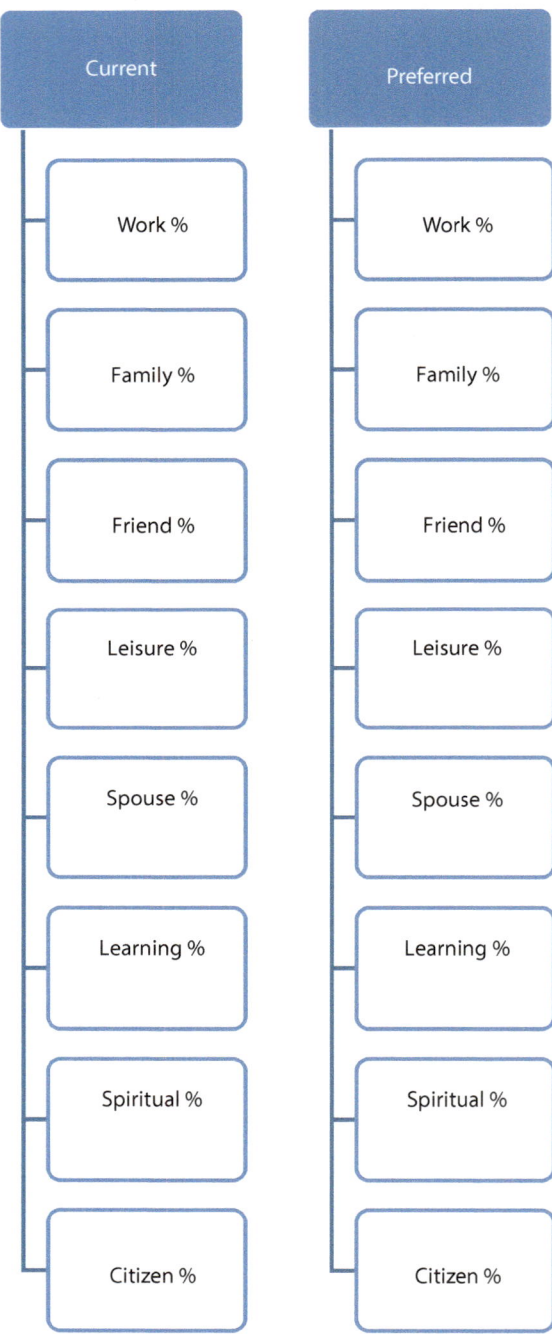

Vignettes
Vignette 1
Nursing is the best job in the world. I began my career with the vision that I would become a forensic scientist. I envisioned working on something that, was of high stature and respect. On my journey, I encountered others who asked me if that was what I wanted to do. They saw something in me that I didn't see in myself. It was a connection with others. They saw a registered nurse (RN) when I did not. They would ask, why do you want to go work in a lab every day with few people around you? Are you sure you would like that? I would say I am not sure, but I like solving things and working through a problem. They would say "consider nursing", you are explaining things every day but with people instead of in a lab, my skill with people was something that they felt would bring me joy. I decided to give it a try, applied, and began school. I quickly found out this career was the perfect combination of solving challenges and bringing out my caring nature with people. Both are hugely rewarding for me. I quickly found myself moving up the career ladder because I was successful, not because I made a lot of money as a registered nurse (RN) but because my soul was doing the work I was born to do.

Vignette 2
What is the hardest thing about being a nurse?
For me, the hardest thing about nursing is the physical side. Being on my feet for an entire 12-hour shift, working night shifts, and lifting patients take a toll. I attend weekly yoga classes and do CrossFit for stamina and endurance. The stronger I am physically, the better I can handle with whatever nursing throws my way.

References

Jacobsen (2015) Boundary Theory, Work/Life Balance, and Mindfulness. Workhuman.com Retrieved from https://www.workhuman.com/resources/globoforce-blog/boundary-theory-work-life-balance-and-mindfulness

Kohll (2018) The evolving definition of work-life balance. Forbes.com Retrieved from https://www.forbes.com/sites/alankohll/2018/03/27/the-evolving-definition-of-work-life-balance/#17463b749ed3

Laskowski (2020) How much should the average adult exercise every day? MayoClinic.org Retrieved from https://www.mayoclinic.org/healthy-lifestyle/fitness/expert-answers/exercise/faq-20057916

Legg (2019) Intrinsic motivation: how to pick up healthy motivation techniques. Healthline. Retrieved from: https://www.healthline.com/health/intrinsic-motivation

McCarthy (2018) Americans wasted 768 million vacation days last year. Forbes. Retrieved from https://www.forbes.com/sites/niallmccarthy/2019/08/19/americans-wasted-768-million-vacation-days-last-year-infographic/#7a322fdf248c

Nurse.com (2020) Nurse writer shares stories from his 32-year career. Retrieved from https://www.nurse.com/blog/2019/03/25/nurse-writer-shares-stories-from-32-year-career/

Robbins (2007) Awaken the Giant Within How to take immediate control of your mental, emotional, physical, and financial destiny. Simon and Schuster

Wolfe (2020) 7 Reasons You can't get motivated today (solutions included!). Themuse.com. Retrieved from: https://www.themuse.com/advice/7-reasons-you-cant-get-motivated-today-solutions-included

Charting YOUR Career Path: External Strategies and Issues

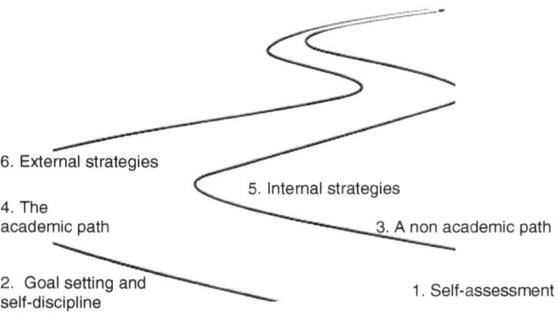

6. External strategies

5. Internal strategies

4. The academic path

3. A non academic path

2. Goal setting and self-discipline

1. Self-assessment

Contents

© Springer Nature Switzerland AG 2020
J. M. Manning, *The Path to Building a Successful Nursing Career*,
https://doi.org/10.1007/978-3-030-50023-8_6

Courage starts with showing up and letting ourselves be seen. —Brene Brown

Know where you want to go and make sure the right people know about it.
—Author unknown

6.1 Networking

Networking—some years back, I remember thinking, what is that? Why is it essential for professional growth? How will it help me get where I want to be? For some, networking is something you do without even realizing you are doing it. Networking is essential in all aspects of your career. If you work in a hospital, you network when you talk with colleagues working in other departments and connect to discuss new processes. These discussions help you perform your job better and result in improved patient care. Networking occurs when you talk with administration about issues in the workplace and inform them of what needs to be addressed. Any interaction where you are connecting with others to help improve the workplace, which impacts you and patient care, is networking on a local level.

These connections extend beyond your place of employment when you network with others, such as in continuing education forums where groups with similar interests talk about common issues and work towards better solutions by sharing their success stories as well as their challenges.

When you are building a successful nursing career, networking can connect you to your next employer or your next school, where you may obtain advanced education.

Some of the top strategies for networking include:

6.1.1 Networking on Social Media

Tips for networking in today's highly technological climate are made easier with social media. Social media consists of websites and applications that enable a user to share or create content or actively participate in social networking. Networking with social media or social networking includes using internet-based social media to connect with others. The purpose can be social, business, or both. Popular social media sites are Facebook, Twitter, LinkedIn, and Instagram. There are many other examples in addition to these. By conducting a Google search, you may connect with an ideal social media site that meets your needs. You have access to many professional resources through social networking. On social media, you can connect with millions of people, find mentors, collaborate or identify future job openings.

Twitter is an American microblogging and social networking service where users post instant messages called "tweets." Users can post, like, or retweet. The hashtag symbol (#) can be added before a relevant keyword in a tweet to categorize the tweet and help show the tweet more efficiently in a Twitter search. By clicking on a hashtagged word, you see other tweets that include the hashtag. Hashtags are an easy way to spot persons with shared interests.

Linkedin is a business and employment service operating from a website or mobile application. This service is geared to professional networking. Here employers can post jobs, and job seekers can post their resumes. Contacts can be shared, and one can optimize a profile. With Linkedin, one can send connection requests to those of influence in a specialty field. Linkedin has mentorship and consulting feature for persons interested in networking.

Facebook is a social media and technology company that helps people connect with friends, families, communities, and businesses. Facebook group is a feature that helps make connections. Groups such as new graduate family registered nurse (RN) practitioner, social nursing resource, nursing leadership, and just about any group related to an area of nursing you are interested in are listed on Facebook groups. You can begin your group as well.

Remember, the key to networking is to build relationships. Introduce yourself and your interests on your site. Complete your bio so others can know your interests. Comment on posts and share resources with the group. You need to be active. This is an inexpensive and highly effective way to connect with others.

6.1.2 Network by Blogging

A blogger primarily creates content that can be used for personal or business use. It can also be used for networking and other professional means. A blog is a discussion website where content is presented in the form of opinions, stories, videos and photos.

A variety of topics are being blogged on any given day. In nursing, there are many blogs worthy of following. For example, Lorry Schoenly is a registered nurse (RN) educator and writer who actively blogs about issues in Correctional Nursing. Elizabeth Scala is an author, speaker, trainer, and Reiki Master. She consults with organizations to help the nursing staff cope with the realities often faced in nursing work. Brittney Wilson is a clinical informatics registered nurse (RN) and blogs on topics related to healthcare. Registered nurse (RN) Nacole is a blogger who aims to help nursing students. There are many more nursing bloggers out there and likely one which is of interest to you and applicable to your career development.

6.1.3 Network by Volunteering

Volunteering is a way to give back to the community or make a difference to the people around you. It can also be an opportunity to develop new skills or building upon current skills and knowledge. For example, the American Red Cross relies on the registered nurses (RNs) and student registered nurses (RNs) to provide relief services around the world. Registered nurses (RNs) work with communities to prepare for disasters, facilitate emergency communication, assist in blood drives, operate immunization sites, and respond to local emergencies. There are other opportunities such as nursing homes and senior care facilities where registered nurses (RNs) assist with events, outings, and visit with the residents. Your local hospital is a great place for volunteering. One can volunteer in specialty areas and obtain insight into what the work environment is like. Other areas where registered nurse (RN) volunteers are needed are community health events and homeless shelters.

6.1.4 Network by Attending Professional Development Conferences

Nursing conferences are a valuable way to boost your career. The larger meetings can be intimidating. It is essential to take the time to plan your attendance and attend as many events as possible. The smaller conference can have as many as 100 attendees; larger conference can have more than 1000. Conferences typically use several strategies to help attendees network. There generally are events that aim to encourage interaction. These can be in the form of a workshop, between session networking, dinners, or evening walking groups. Attendee contact information is usually shared among all participants. Talk to colleagues in your area to find out which conferences are recommended. Meetings are also a great place to learn about the newest practice trends and updates in practice. Top registered nurses (RNs) in the field are often there. An exhibit hall is a place where vendors display the newest products in practice. Also, organizations are available to answer questions about membership and the benefits of membership. Conferences are a great place to obtain continuing education credits.

Successful attendance requires advanced planning, as one typically cannot attend all sessions. Register early to receive the best discounts. Print out any necessary materials before attending. If you have business cards, bring them. If not, bring contact information you can easily share. Identify which sessions you want to visit before the conference begins. Prepare to walk a lot if the meeting is large. Bring something for note-taking, e.g., notebook and a pen and download the conference application if available for your smart phone. ► Case Example 6.1 describes tips for getting the most out of a meeting or conference.

> **Case Example 6.1 Tips for Getting the Most Out of a Meeting or Conference**
>
> Tips for getting the most out of a conference:
> - Attend three meetings before deciding to join a group. The first meeting is to overcome fear, the second is to learn about it, and the third is to determine if you like it
> - Introduce yourself by giving your first and last name. Say something about yourself to get the conversation going. Even people that know you well or met you before can have temporary forgetfulness with names
> - Wear comfortable shoes and clothes, be prepared for standing for long periods
> - Wear your name tag on the right side, so people see it when you shake hands
> - Plan your conversations on time. Come prepared with small talk
> - Keep business cards handy, use them to leave a tangible reminder of who you are
> - Relax and try to enjoy yourself. If you are uncomfortable, find a person who looks nervous and tries to set them at ease
>
> Diamani (2014)

6.1.5 **Signature Look at Events**

» I can live for two months on a good compliment —Unknown

Style is one strategy in creating a personal brand. Your style should empower you to take on the world each day. Consider "your look." Do you have a "go-to" style when dressing for a professional gathering? Consider which elements of your outfit are signature for you? Maybe a style of dress or pants with a jacket Or possibly a specific color? If you need to design a signature look, consider the following: What outfit looks best with your body shape? You do not need to be able to wear any style. Do you have certain outfits where you received compliments? Do you record your best outfits as a strategy for future purchases?

Does another's style inspire you? Find some common themes you want to borrow for your signature look. Keep your go-to clothes in one section of your closet. A personal theme or brand can be a time saver when you are in a hurry. Remember, it doesn't matter what type of job you have; style is part of the way you dress. Do you have a signature item? Possibly a piece of jewelry or color lipstick.

6.1.6 **Ask for a Connection**

Asking for a connection is as simple as it sounds. You need to be courageous and consider that everyone wants to network with those who have similar interests.

6.1.7 **Create Networking Cards**

The next step is considering how to connect. You can use business cards. Another strategy is to connect via LinkedIn. Taking a picture of the contact information is also helpful.

A networking card should include (◨ Fig. 6.1):
- Your full name with middle initial
- Credentials
- Title
- Address
- Email address

◨ **Fig. 6.1**   Networking card

Jane S. Doe RN, BSN

Staff Registered nurse (RN)

1234 Parkway Ave

jdoe@organization.com

twitter URL

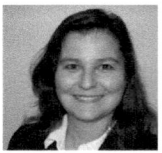

- Phone number
- Social media URL
- Picture of you and your organization's brand
- Take a snapshot of your networking card to share when you do not have paper copies with you.

6.1.8 Be Ahead of the Curve

Networking is about being up to date. Through your exposure to professional development and reading information online on your professional organization website, you are setting yourself up for success in understanding the status of the rapidly changing healthcare landscape. Having current knowledge allows you to discuss trends for the future expertly. Do not think you need to know everything, bring the information you have to the conversation, listen to understand when interacting with others. From there, you can work together when discussing important topics (Nurse.org 2020; Hewlett 2014).

6.2 Professional Organization Membership and Participation

There are many benefits to professional organization membership. Professional organizations expose members to some essential aspects of nursing practice. One of the most common benefits is providing the most up-to-date information in a specialty area. This information may be the most recent research or the most updated policy changes. The most common issues are addressed with solutions to problems (► Case Example 6.2).

Case Example 6.2 Top Reasons to Join a Professional Organization

1. Professional development
2. Networking
3. Discounts
4. Committees
5. Staying up to date
6. Career assistance
7. Grants and scholarships

6.2.1 Professional Development

Professional organizations offer professional development, usually for continuing education credits, which are essential for professional growth. Continuing education is typically free to members or deeply discounted. Some nursing organizations have an official journal that publishes the most up-to-date peer-reviewed articles, research, evidence-based practice, and practice guidelines. Usually, professional development is free to members. The topics are relevant, up to date, and often presented by experts in the field.

6.2.2 Networking

Networking is another benefit of professional organization membership. Member contact information is shared and can be accessed by fellow members. Online forums, networking events, annual conferences, and local meetings are typically available for members. Advocacy groups may be available in the profession for different areas in nursing. For example, the American Association of Critical Care Nurses offers resources and advocacy for new nurses, experienced nurses, and nurse managers.

6.2.3 Discounts

Discounts for conferences are available for members. Most large organizations have annual meetings that bring members together to network and learn about timely topics. Membership may offer other benefits such as discounts on services such as nursing malpractice insurance, cell phone service, life insurance, travel agents, and certifications. Discounts for the organization's journal may be available as well as annual conference discounts.

6.2.4 Committees

Membership offers the opportunity to join a committee with a specific focus. For example, the American Nurses Association (ANA) has countless committees, task forces, or groups who work to promote the profession of nursing. If you are interested in influencing health policy, the ANA publishes position statements on important policy topic areas such as access to healthcare and support for immunizations. Members can provide feedback on position statements or join a committee involved in writing position statements. You can apply to join one of the committees, and the competition for being selected varies depending on the type of group.

6.2.5 Staying Up to Date

Members can stay up to date with news and changes in a specialized area of nursing practice. Members can develop a broader knowledge base and perspective. Information can be disseminated via the website, organizational blogs, journals, books, etc.

6.2.6 Career Assistance

Members can often access assistance with career growth via job postings and mentorship programs. Information about the job search, salaries, benefits, job descriptions is often described. For example, the American Nurses Association offers an 8-month mentorship program for members with mentors nationwide. Also, the

American Association of Colleges of Nursing provides a career center with job positions, career development resources, salary information, vacancy information, and fact sheets on nationwide job positions.

6.2.7 Grants and Scholarships

Some professional organizations provide grants and scholarships for members. For example, the American Organization for Nursing Leadership (AONL) offers research grants for members interested in researching topics of interest to nursing leaders. The National Student Nurses Association (NSNA) provides scholarships to students studying nursing.

The benefits of a professional organization may vary greatly, and members need to take the time to learn about the many available benefits to maximize the money spent on membership. Most members do not take advantage of all the benefits available to them.

6.3 Work Environments

Nursing work is demanding. The hours are long with high stress and changing conditions. Decisions made by nurses have significant implications for the health and lives of the patients served. Patients are sick and stressed. Nurses interact with patients who are not at their best. The work is fast-paced, intense, and dynamic. Quick responses are needed, and there are many demands. Shortages complicate the situation, and many units are chronically understaffed and experience high turnover. New nurses are continually entering the workforce. The 12-h shifts afford more days each week, but the schedule on the workdays are grueling, and there is little time for self-care. A 12 h shift can quickly stretch too much longer considering paperwork and commuting. There is physical and mental strain. Nurses go home with little energy and time to care for themselves or others in the home.

On another note, nurses are resilient and able to deal with stress in a thriving healthcare work environment. The work environment has become more of a topic of conversation especially during the pandemic.

The AACN (2020) defines a healthy work environment (HWE) as an interrelated system of people, structures, and practices enabling registered nurses (RNs) to engage in work processes. AACN describes six standards of a healthy work environment (◘ Fig. 6.2). They include skilled communication, true collaboration, effective decision-making, appropriate staffing, meaningful recognition, and authentic leadership (AACN 2016).

6.3.1 Skilled Communication

Skilled communication is described as an open and productive conversation among those on the healthcare team resulting in optimal patient outcomes. Collaboration is encouraged through qualified discussion. Organizations that support skilled

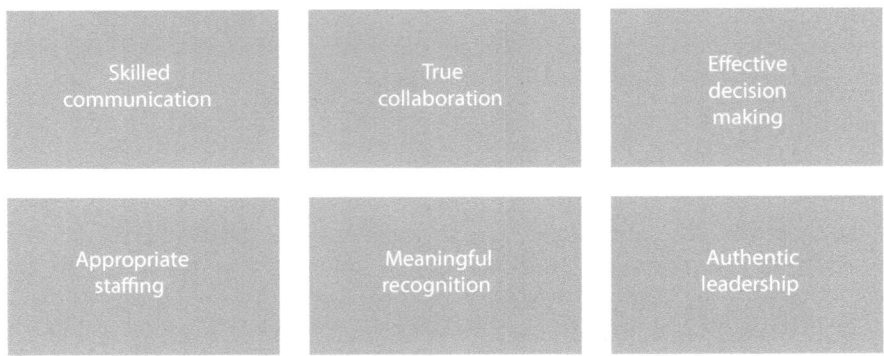

6

◘ Fig. 6.2   AACN healthy work environment standards (American Association of Critical-Care Nurses 2020)

communication encourage the respective sharing of information. Nurses who are experienced in communication can find solutions that result in optimal patient outcomes.

6.3.2 True Collaboration

The true collaboration consists of successful teamwork and a supportive environment where practice is developed. Nurses are afforded decision-making authority and are provided resources to support the achievement of the common goal of promoting optimal patient outcomes. Healthcare team members work together as equal partners in fostering collaboration.

6.3.3 Effective Decision-Making

Effective decision-making empowers nurses by ensuring they have a voice during decision-making processes and are involved in designing protocols that benefit both staff and patients. Organizations must ensure decision-making is deliberate and respects the rights of all to participate in decision-making and evaluating the outcome of decisions.

6.3.4 Appropriate Staffing

Appropriate staffing includes the use of staffing models that meets the needs of the organization, nurses, and patients. The nurse skill mix must be matched with patient needs. Nurses should be part of the development of effective staffing models and must obtain skills and competence in understanding the organizational staffing processes.

6.3.5 Meaningful Recognition

Meaningful recognition includes the recognition of the healthcare team members and the value they bring to the organization. A recognition system should be incorporated into the hospital's processes, and everyone plays a role in recognition programs.

6.3.6 Authentic Leadership

Nurse leaders embrace the healthy work environment standards to ensure a cohesive work environment that elevates patient care outcomes. Leaders must develop their skills and work toward a culture where all elements of the healthy work environment are upheld and effectively implemented.

6.4 Nurse Work Environment Expectations

According to the Bureau of Labor Statistics (BLS), nurses' duties include recording medical histories, patient symptoms, administration of treatments, setting up a patient plan of care, observing patients, recording assessment information, consulting with the healthcare team members, operating and monitoring medical equipment, and other similar duties (Campbellsville University 2020).

>> We make a living by what we get, we make a life by what we give. —Winston Churchill

6.5 Mentors

A mentor is a trusted adviser who typically guides a less experienced person through modeling and advisement. The role of a mentor is to share information about his or her career path. There are eight elements of mentorship: coaching, support, goal setting, training, motivation, advisement, success, and direction (◘ Fig. 6.3). Through coaching, training, advisement, and support, the mentee can put initiatives into place, which results in performance improvement and "unlock" potential. Goal setting and direction are used to quantify objectives the mentee wishes to achieve. The coach aims to motivate the mentee during the mentorship process. Mentors can be an invaluable tool when exploring careers, setting goals, identifying resources, and developing contacts on the path to building a successful nursing career.

6.5.1 Formal Mentor

A formal mentor is one who assists the mentee because of an official role or agreement. Persons participating in mentorship programs can be formal mentors where there is an agreement with set guidelines for the mentor/mentee relationship. Typically a formal mentor is linked with a mentee through an agreement. During the initial

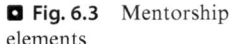

■ **Fig. 6.3** Mentorship elements

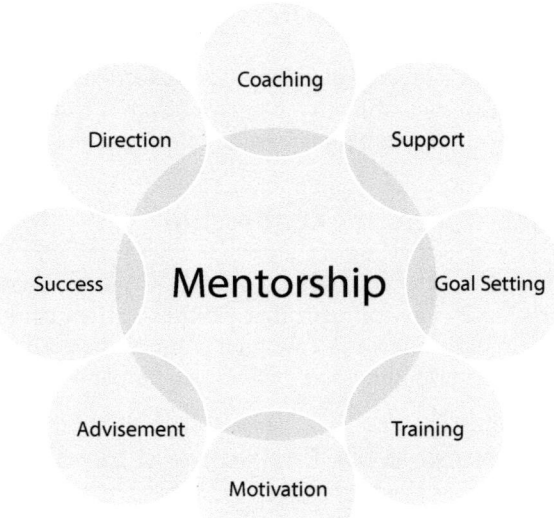

■ **Table 6.1**   Obtaining feedback

Get focused	Ensure you are not distracted by other issues and provide full attention to the information you are receiving
Allow adequate time	Schedule enough time so you can listen and not rush. Reflect on the information as you hear it is key to understanding
Understand the feedback	Seek clarification or ask for information to be repeated if you are unclear
Ask for guidance	If feedback indicates a need to change behavior, seek advice or directions for change. Ask for outcomes which will show a successful behavioral change
Show appreciation	Feedback is useful information. Thank the person providing it
Think about feedback	Evaluate behavior in light of the new information. Reflect on implications and consider changes

phase of the relationship, goals are set. Ongoing meetings are scheduled to discuss progress towards a mutually agreed-upon goal, which helps the mentee advance their career. The mentor is responsible for serving as a role model, providing feedback, and linking the mentee to information that supports their goals. At the end of the formal relationship, success in achievement of objectives is evaluated, and the relationship ends or continues based on a mutual agreement between mentor and mentee.

A mentor can assist with an evaluation of performance and serve as a social mirror. Feedback is the information we receive from others about the impact of our behavior. It allows us to view ourselves from another perspective. Riley (2004) recommends the following steps when soliciting feedback (■ Table 6.1).

6.5.2 Informal Mentor

Informal mentors do not provide mentorship in a formal role. They informally guide the mentee in a casual way where there are no set guidelines. An informal mentor is someone who interacts with the mentee ongoingly. Challenges are discussed, and feedback is provided. The informal mentor serves as an unbiased sounding board for the mentee to share with confidence. The mentor offers feedback based on their experience and perspective.

Mentees and mentors benefit from formal and informal relationships with mentors. Anyone working on building their career is recommended to seek both formal and informal mentorship relationships. Both are helpful on the path to build a successful nursing career.

Strategies
Complete these free online quizzes:

Learn to network through these eight tips. *Forbes.* ▶ https://www.forbes.com/sites/theyec/2014/07/28/how-to-network-the-right-way-eight-tips/#453222206d47

American Nurses Association: Join a mentorship program. ▶ https://www.nursingworld.org/membership/member-benefits/professional-development-resources/

❓ Activities
— Use your journal to answer the following questions:
  1. Reflection: do you have the courage to receive honest feedback? Do you have the courage to give honest feedback to a friend or colleague? How do you respond to negative feedback?
  2. Create a list of those you look up to. Can any of these persons serve as an informal mentor?
  3. Review the websites of several organizations you are interested in. If you are not familiar with organizations available, write down what areas of nursing you are interested in. Then search for nursing organizations using the keywords you have identified. Conduct a search for an organization. Identify the benefits of the organization. Consider joining one which best meets your interest, needs, and budget.
  4. Create a profile on LinkedIn. Add a bio, professional picture. Explore contacts and ask to connect with them. Aim high, connect with those at the pinnacle of their careers, and serving in a level you would aim for in your long-term goals.
  5. Reflect on your current work environment. What are some good and not so good aspects? Review the six healthy work environment standards. Determine which ones can be improved. Discuss some strategies for improvement with your supervisor.
  6. Define your mission statement. In 140 characters, sum up your strengths, passions, and interests. If you have 30–60 s with someone, how would you sell yourself? Your words should be authentic and confidently express yourself. Seek to define yourself based on your brand rather than your title.

6

Vignettes
Vignette 1
What keeps you working at your current job?

I'm impressed with the work environment here, and the collaborative spirit of of the team. Just by sitting in the waiting room, it's clear to me that this healthcare organization has a patient-first priority. I'm eager to work with people who are passionate about providing quality care.

Vignette 2
Ten things I wish I had known earlier in my nursing career:

Fairley (2019) 10 things I wish I had known early in my nursing career. Capella University. Retrieved from: ► https://www.capella.edu/blogs/cublog/capella-nursing-faculty-member-shares-10-tips-for-nurses/

Collaborate: Sometimes, nurses hesitate to work with other disciplines. They may choose to try and handle a situation by themselves. However, all disciplines can offer ideas to assist the profession as well as benefit patient care. Collaboration can have a positive influence on the quality of care in a variety of healthcare settings.

Be resilient: In nursing, change happens daily. You may be moved to a different floor or be unexpectedly asked to work with a different type of patient. It's essential to be flexible, even in the face of challenges, and keep a positive attitude. Nurse leaders often look for nurses who are flexible. It means that you can be counted on to take on new and different opportunities in the organization.

Explore nursing: It's easy to stay the course without exploring more of the field. Learn about each aspect of this varied and dynamic career. For instance, find out how finance or health policy relates to nursing. Stay current in nursing trends through blogs and professional organizations. You might be surprised at the variety of opportunities you find within your nursing career.

Learn the business of healthcare: At the start of my career, I worked as a staff nurse at a hospital and went many years without getting a raise. I saw new hospital buildings being built, technology investments, and didn't understand why the hospital could afford to expand, but not give me a higher salary. My nurse manager explained that the nursing budget was different from the hospital budget. That was my introduction to the business of healthcare and the realization that understanding the business aspects of nursing was essential to my career development.

Pay attention to political nursing issues: Learning more about health politics will open your mind to the professional challenges nurses face. As a nurse, learn about the legislative process and regulations. Keep up to date on political changes. If you don't know, find out about how new policies impact change by attending legislative meetings, conferences, and webinars that deal with political issues concerning healthcare.

Get a mentor: I believe every nurse needs to have a mentor, especially young nurses. It is essential to have someone you can talk to. I found my mentors through observation. I looked at them and thought, "I want to be just like them someday." It's not about who has the most experience; it's about the mentor that can provide the best experience to a mentee. Seek out someone approachable and who inspires you to be the best you can be.

Find opportunities for professional development: Always make sure you have opportunities for professional development, for example, attending conferences or joining a professional organization. Opportunities to get involved may not be obvious. The only way to learn is to network and ask questions. When you use specific methods and strategies to deliver best practices to patients, the outcomes are usually very positive. So why not invest in learning best practices?

Seek community involvement: Get outside the walls of the hospital. What's happening in the community is where you can pick up new ideas and bring that knowledge back to your organization. Volunteering with diverse populations in the community will expand your knowledge and skills in working with different patient populations in your healthcare setting.

Invest in continuing education: No matter your age now, is the time to invest in expanding your knowledge and career. Nursing is a lifelong career, and development is vital. To avoid stagnation in your career, it's essential to invest in continuing education.

Further, your education: There are now so many avenues a nurse can take, but you can't advance your position unless you have advanced training, certifications, or both. Growing professions in nursing often require an advanced degree. It doesn't matter if you've been a nurse for 20 years; you still need to advance your education to get ahead in your career (Beale 2016; Schneider 2020).

» Many people put pressure on themselves and think it will be way toov hard for them to live out their dreams. A mentor is there to say it is not that tough and not as hard as you think. —Joe Jonas

» Show me a successful individual, and I will show you someone who had real positive influences in his or her life. I don't care what you do for a living if you do it well I am sure someone was cheering you on or showing the way. A mentor—Denzel Washington

References

American Association of Critical-Care Nurses (AACN) (2020) Healthy work environment standard. https://www.aacn.org/nursing-excellence/aacn-standards

Beale K (2016) Mentoring new nurses. Am J Nurs 116(10):13. https://journals.lww.com/ajnonline/Fulltext/2016/10000/Mentoring_New_Registerednurse_(RN)s.3.aspx

Campbellsville University (2020) What to expect: work environment for nurses. https://online.campbellsville.edu/program-resources/work-environment-for-nurses/

Diamani H (2014) How to attend a conference like a bootstrapped entrepreneur. CreateSpace Independent Publishing, Scotts Valley

Hewlett SA (2014) Executive presence: the missing link between merit and success. HarperAudio, New York

Nurse.org (2020) 10 networking tips for nurses who hate networking. https://nurse.org/articles/tips-for-nurse-networking

Schneider A (2020) Nursing organizations: the role they play in professional development. RN.com. https://www.rn.com/nursing-organizations-the-role-they-play-in-professional-development/

The Basics of Professional Growth

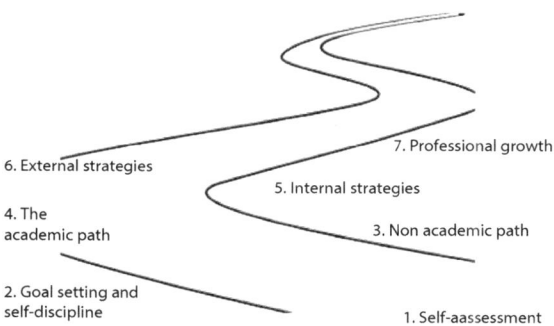

Contents

© Springer Nature Switzerland AG 2020
J. M. Manning, *The Path to Building a Successful Nursing Career*,
https://doi.org/10.1007/978-3-030-50023-8_7

Healthy work environments cannot live with distrust nor without civility. —*Unknown*

Hate begets hate; violence begets violence; toughness begets a greater toughness.
We must meet the forces of hate with the power of love. —*Martin Luther King Jr.*

7.1 First, Be Kind

» Three things in life are essential, the first is to be kind, the second is to be kind, and the third is to be kind. —Henry James

Has anyone ever told you that kindness matters? I bet you are thinking, of course, kindness matters. In work environments, kindness is an underrated quality. In nursing work environments, compassion and individualized care are essential to calming patients and strengthening registered nurse (RN)–patient relationships, which ultimately improve outcomes. Kindness is one of the most powerful therapeutic interventions. In a world of highly scientific intervention, the most basic, nontechnical action—kindness is the key to success in the healthcare field.

7.1.1 Jean Watson: Theory of Human Caring®

Jean Watson, a registered nurse (RN) theorist, described a caring science theory that begins with loving-kindness as a primary value of the registered nurse (RN)–patient relationship. Her theory includes ten carative factors and transpersonal caring relationship core principles. The carative factors emphasize the cultivation of sensitivity to one's self and others and the development of a helping-trusting relationship with patients. The core principles of Watson's Theory of Human Caring Science include (◘ Fig. 7.1):

- The practice of loving-kindness and equanimity (inner balance)
  - Caring starts with caring for oneself
- Authentic presence
  - Enabling an internal belief system
- Cultivation of one's spiritual practice toward wholeness of mind/body/spirit
  - Moving beyond ego to wholeness of body, mind, and spirit
- Being in a caring-healing environment
  - Ensuring presence in a supportive environment
- Allowing miracles by being open to the unexpected
  - Open to events that are not rationale or easy to understand

The core concepts of her theory are founded in a relational caring for self and others. Her theory was initially based on the registered nurse (RN)–patient relationship. In recent years, her theory has been expanded to include human to human relationships and can be applied in the healthcare workplace. When caring is expressed between and among professionals, a transpersonal (between humans), intentional (purposeful), and transcendent (uplifting) dynamic occurs, which impacts the entire system. Expressing compassion and kindness for others in the

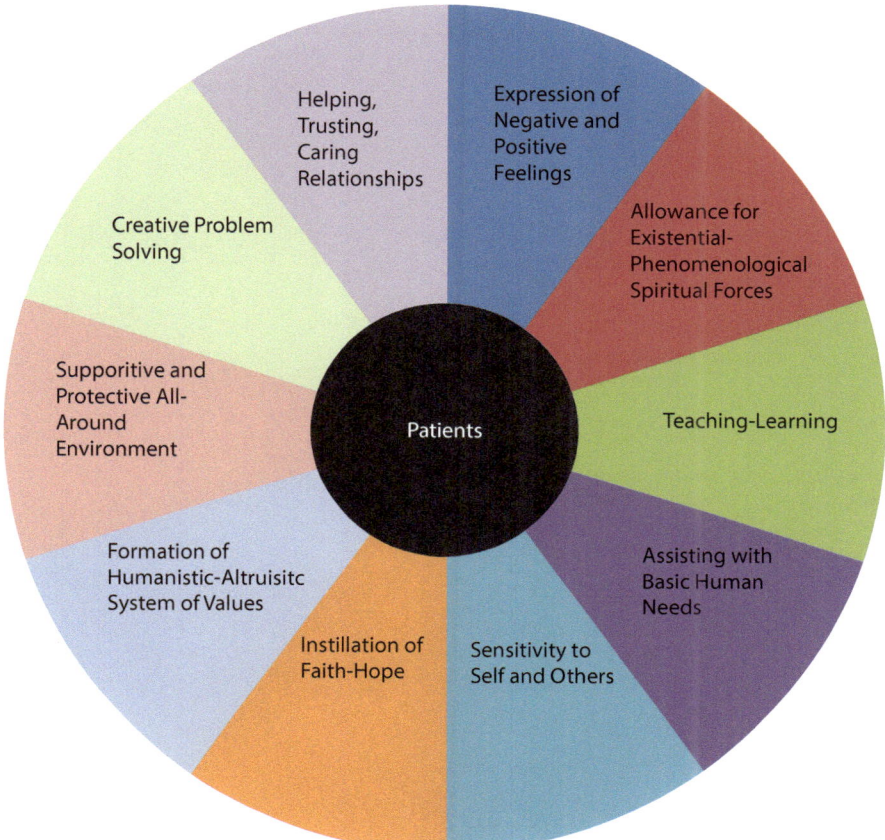

☐ **Fig. 7.1** Watson ten caritas processes of transpersonal caring theory (Wei and Watson 2019; Watson 2011)

workplace cultivates a sense of belonging and is a foundation of workplace culture which impacts patient care quality. The result is a feeling of joy in work in complex healthcare work environments (Wei and Watson 2019).

» Kindness and empathy are key to communication.

Unfortunately, kindness sometimes gets lost in nursing. The reasons this happens may be due to the fast work pace, emotional care that is given to patients, variation in the availability of resources, and registered nurse (RN) burnout. The result is poor patient care, poor work environments, and worse, poor patient outcomes.

Similar to other positive personality characteristics, kindness is partially innate and partially intentional. Some people are naturally kind; others must intentionally work on demonstrating kindness even in the most challenging of circumstances. Showing kindness can be done in nursing work environments using simple strategies. Strategies that aim to promote kindness in work environments are described in ► Case Example 7.1.

Case Example 7.1 Strategies to Demonstrate Kindness in Work Environments

- Make a fresh pot of coffee
- Clean the microwave
- Make a promise not to speak negatively about a colleague
- Write a thank-you note
- Smile
- Say thank you
- Buy a co-worker a snack or lunch
- Give kudos
- Organize a charity drive
- Organize a volunteer day

7

□ **Fig. 7.2**   Keltner's survival of the kindest

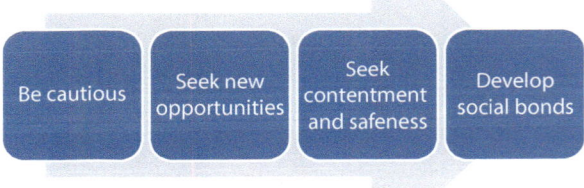

Dacher Keltner, a Professor of Psychology at the University of California, coined a phrase, "survival of the kindest." This phrase is based on major emotional regulation systems or survival instincts that drive human behaviors (□ Fig. 7.2). The first is the avoidance system operated by our brain's negativity bias. This instinctual system encourages us to be cautious and avoid danger. The second system is the achievement system where we are driven to see new opportunities in life, or "carrots." The third instinct guides how we approach our world. When we do not need to defend ourselves to avoid danger and resources are available (not just struggling to survive), we developed a sense of contentment and safeness. We begin to look outwards, beyond survival needs, and connect in a harmonious way allowing us to become kinder to ourselves and others. Social bonds are encouraged as opposed to competition. One person can start changing their behavior, and ripple effects can follow.

There is a long-held belief that humans are wired to be selfish. A wide range of studies have collected evidence to show humans become more compassionate and collaborative along our journey to survive. Keltner's research has supported the survival of humans have evolved the capability to provide care to those in need, Cooperation and sympathy is one of our strongest instincts (University of California, Berkeley 2009).

Studies on kindness have demonstrated a substantial impact on physical and mental health. For example, volunteerism, which is done out of selflessness, is a stronger predictor of longevity in life than physical health, smoking, gender, and marital status (Kahl 2019). The belief is that by helping others, positive emotions are evoked which fight the adverse effects of stress. Additional tips on practicing kindness and encouraging connections with others in the workplace are described in ▶ Case Example 7.2 (Kahl 2019).

Case Example 7.2 Tips on Practicing Kindness and Encouraging Connection with Others

Some tips for practicing kindness and encouraging connection with others in the workplace include:

- Slow down when coming into work, say good morning or hello to colleagues often, smile
- Smile every day for one week and notice what happens and how you feel
- Consider others, change the water in the water cooler, don't leave the coffee empty, ask others if they want coffee when you get some
- Vocalize your praise of others. Compliment a colleague for a week and notice the effect it has on you
- Ask others, "how are you?", stop and listen. Notice if others are under stress or feeling ill or getting behind
- Make time to write a thank-you note to a colleague and show appreciation
- Take time at the end of a meeting to highlight positives. Show application for others in meetings
- Wish someone well at work. Seize a moment with another employee to wish them a good day. Notice how this affects you
- Be a cheerleader for something or someone and put in a positive comment when others are gossiping

---

These tips lead to not only impact others but yourself. These tips also do not take a lot of time or energy. They do not cost anything. These tips make the workplace more meaningful and productive. They encourage productivity. Kindness boosts your well-being and gives you a deeper purpose in the workplace. Kindness week is February 10th–16th; it is a great time to boost morale in the workplace with kind initiatives. The initiatives should continue year-round.

7.2 Civility

What is Civility and Incivility?

Civility is defined as formal politeness and courtesy in behavior or speech. The term civility comes from the Latin word "citizen" and refers to civilized conduct. In 2015, the American nurses Association (ANA) released a position statement regarding the roles and responsibilities of registered nurse (RNs) to promote and sustain workplace cultures which are free of incivility, bullying, and violence. The ANA code of ethics states registered nurses (RNs) are required to "create an ethical environment and culture of civility and kindness, treating colleagues, coworkers, employees, students, and others with dignity and respect" (ANA 2015, p. 4).

What Does Incivility Look Like?

In the workplace, incivility, bullying, and workplace violence contribute to a phenomenon of harmful actions occurring in the workplace. Graphic displays of aggressive acts, incivility, or failing to take action when action is warranted are to no longer be tolerated. Harmful actions come in the form of overt, demeaning comments, or intimidation between coworkers. Other acts may be less apparent and include failing to intervene or withholding vital information. The overall range of actions related to this phenomenon has impacted nursing negatively and, in some cases, is accepted and condoned.

What is the Impact of Incivility?

Registered nurses (RNs) who experience these events firsthand understand the detrimental effects. They have experienced a lack of understanding from others, and their experiences have not been taken seriously. The harmful effects accumulate and are additive burdens on the organization. There is a perception of a "culture of silence," fear of retaliation, and an understanding that "nothing will change." Ultimately, the impact on the profession is severed and an active role in driving cultural change to end incivility, bullying, and violence in the workplace is needed.

Understanding incivility, bullying, and workplace violence are essential in transitioning to a culture of respect, safety, and effective communication in the workplace. Incivility includes rude behaviors such as gossiping, spreading rumors, and refusing to assist another employee. The use of condescending tones, public criticism, and name-calling are examples of incivility. These behaviors can occur feel to face, via email or other online forms. Those targeted, as well as bystanders, felt the impact. If left unaddressed, the situation can progress. Bullying is a repeated and unwanted harmful action that aims to humiliate, offend, or distress another employee. Sanctions include undermining, degrading, and harming the individual. Examples include hostile remarks, verbal attacks, threats, taunts, and intimidation. The actions increase can increase in frequency and intensity. The impact is lasting physical and psychological difficulties for the recipient of the bullying.

Bullying aims to create defenselessness and injustice upon another. It can occur at all levels of the organization and in any direction. Aggression, which ostracizes, marginalizes or expels the individual from the group, is an example of bullying. When more than one person commits the act which harms or eliminates a targeted individual is bullying. The term for bullying in the workplace by more than one individual is referred to as workplace mobbing.

Workplace violence is the physical and psychological actions occurring in the workplace. It includes verbal or physical threats by any person in the workplace. Examples include written or verbal threats, physical or verbal harassment, and homicide. Studies have concluded that up to 24% of respondents have been physically assaulted by a person in the workplace while at work. The impact on the individual is severe, leading to emotional distress, injury, or even death. There are four types of healthcare workplace violence. Type I is where individuals with criminal intent have no relationship with the organization. Type II is where the individual has a relationship with the organization and becomes violent while receiving care. Type III is where employees attack or threaten each other. Type IV is where individuals have interpersonal relationships with the target of the violence but no relation to the organization.

The impact of incivility, bullying, and workplace violence is detrimental to nursing resulting in registered nurses (RN) leaving their job or the profession. There is reduced job satisfaction, personal health, and productivity (Clark 2013).

Respectful relationships need to be valued and recognized in organizations. Safe work environments promote well-being. When employees do not feel safe, the outcomes of the organization suffer. Knowledge regarding this issue is critical. A commitment by RNs in creating a safe and trusting work environment is needed with a shared commitment to dignity and respect. A culture of health and safety results in safe environments for registered nurses (RNs) to provide high-quality care to patients. Employers must ensure work environments are healthy and safe. If not upheld, the organization can be sanctioned according to the Occupational Safety and Health Act (American Nurses Association 2015).

Dr. Cynthia Clark, a registered nurse (RN) theorist, is a registered nurse (RN) known for her extensive work incivility in nursing. Clark created a framework for fostering civility, which is based on a continuum of behaviors (◘ Fig. 7.3). The framework depicts incivility on a continuum from low to high risk. As the risk increases the disruptive behaviors also increase to more threatening and violent behaviors. As a registered nurse (RN) aiming to build our careers, we are responsible for ensuring the workplace is free of incivility, bullying, and workplace violence.

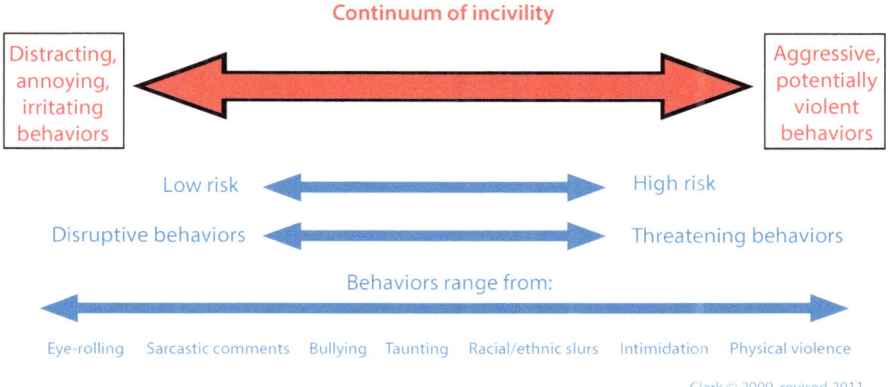

◘ **Fig. 7.3** Clark continuum of incivility (Tillman 2020)

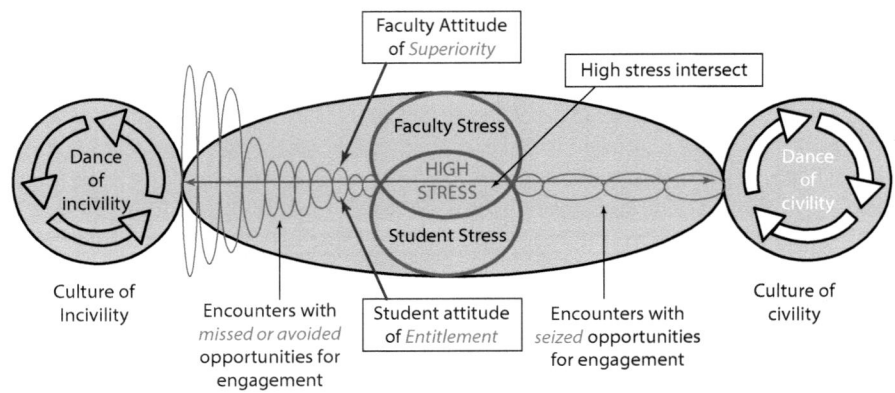

Fig. 7.4 Clark conceptual model for fostering civility (Clark 2020)

Clark developed a similar model to depict incivility in nursing education. In the center, a midpoint shows where high levels of faculty and student stress overlap. When high levels of faculty and student stress occur, with attitudes of student entitlement and faculty superiority and cultures of civility are in jeopardy of becoming uncivil (■ Fig. 7.4).

The conceptual model for fostering civility includes several theoretical areas. The model depicts when high stress intersects between colleagues, encounters result in missed opportunities for engagement. The dance of civility and incivility occurs following intersections of stress between colleagues.

Incivility includes a mixture of harmful actions taken and not taken. Some activities can be overt and include demeaning comments or intimidation to undermine colleagues. Other activities may be less obvious such as failing to intervene or withholding vital informants when actions are indicated and needed. Incivility has touched far too many registered nurses (RNs) over time. When building your nursing career, it is essential to understand the concept and the role you play in promoting or diminishing it.

There are many forms of incivility and include rudeness or discourteous actions, gossiping, spreading rumors, or refusing to assist another colleague. Each of these violates professional standards and diminishes the dignity of the colleague. The effects are far-reaching and impact not only the person targeted but peers, stakeholders, and organizations.

When incivility re-occurs with the intent to humiliate and offend, it is bullying. It may come in the form of hostile remarks, verbal attacks, threats, taunting, intimidation, and refusing support. This action is a safety concern to all in healthcare with lasting physical and psychological implications. It creates feelings of defenselessness and injustice and undermines the right to dignity.

As a person interested in advancing their career, understanding of this behavior is essential, as well as an understanding of strategies and the role one must play in diminishing and eliminating it in the workplace.

How to Improve Civility?

A culture of respect should consistently exist in the workplace. The American Nurses Association code of ethics is a helpful tool for identifying the behaviors needed to ensure you are on the right track in curbing this egregious behavior in the workplace. Ensure environments are safe and promote physical and psychological well-being. Commit to promoting dignity and respect is vital. Legally, employers must provide safe and healthy workplaces for employees.

Some helpful behaviors which support civility include:

- Use clear communication verbally, nonverbally, and in writing (including social media).
- Treat others with respect, dignity, collegiality, and kindness.
- Consider how personal words and actions affect others.
- Avoid gossip and spreading rumors.
- Rely on facts and not conjecture.
- Collaborate and share information where appropriate.
- Provide help when needed, and, if refused, accept refusal gracefully.
- Take responsibility and be accountable for one's actions.
- Recognize that abuse of power or authority is never acceptable.
- Speak directly to the person with whom one has an issue.
- Demonstrate openness to other points of view, perspectives, experiences, and ideas.
- Be polite and respectful and apologize when indicated.
- Encourage, support, and mentor others including new registered nurses (RNs) and experienced registered nurses (RNs).
- Listen to others with interest and respect (Clark 2010).

7.3 Burnout

Burnout is a physical, mental, and emotional state caused by chronic overwork and a sustained lack of job fulfillment and support. It is an exhaustive state.

Nursing work is a high demand job. Shortages consistently persist. Many registered nurses (RNs) work with less than what they need. Stressful situations are frequent. All registered nurses (RNs) are susceptive to burnout. The impact leads to personal and work challenges and can lead to resignation (Waddill-Goad 2016).

Compson (2015) explored the causes and symptoms of burnout. She evaluated burnout within the context of the CARE heuristic, where C = Compassion, A = Awareness, R = Resilient Responding, and E = Empowerment. Each of these approaches aim to help nurses protect themselves against burnout or treat existing symptoms of burnout. Compassion is the ability to open to "the reality of suffering and aspire to its healing." Awareness is knowledge available about what is happening. These include situational, mindful, and self-awareness. Resilience is the ability to maintain function and well-being in the face of stress and adversity. Empowerment is a sense of lowered personal efficacy. It is the perception of professional autonomy, access to resources, ability to influence work decisions in a manner that is consistent with personal values (Compson 2015).

Work-related issues such as exposure to patient death on a regular base, the emotional strain of losing patients, assisting with grieving family members can become overwhelming. The long work hours can also lead to exhaustion and stress. Registered nurses (RNs) in high-stress environments are more susceptible to burnout.

The social environment of nursing can also cause burnout. Nursing is a collaborative field, and the constant pressure to meet social expectations can lead to mental exhaustion. A study examining RNs' reasons for entering the field concluded that those aiming to "help others" may be more susceptible to burnout when they perceive job-related success or failure in a personal way.

Oncology and emergency nursing areas are the highest susceptible areas for burnout. Oncology registered nurses (RNs) form relationships with patients. The emotional journey with them can lead a registered nurse (RN) to feel lost, especially when the patient dies. In the ER where urgency is ongoing, and the pressure is high with large numbers of patients, registered nurses (RNs) are susceptible to burnout in this fast-past entremets.

Burnout symptoms include physical or emotional exhaustion, job-related cynicism, and a low sense of personal accomplishment. If untreated, burnout can lead to clinical depression and compounding of symptoms over time (◘ Fig. 7.5).

Reactions to stress can be physical, emotional, or environmental. The manifestation can become apparent in many ways. Recognition of symptoms may come from yourself or another colleague. The symptoms may become evident in varying intensity.

Early recognition is vital. Common symptoms include irritability. Typically, irritability is chronic and is the first sign. Frequent frustrations become more and more common. Another symptom is persistent calling in sick. When missed days

◘ **Fig. 7.5** Burnout and areas of work life theoretical model (areas of work life are in the outer circles and burnout symptoms are in the inner circles) (Compson 2015)

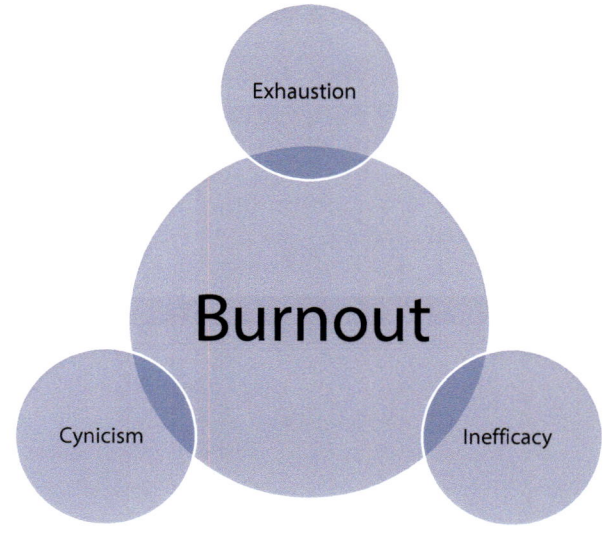

become more prevalent, self-care is often needed. Intolerance to change and a reluctance to adjust is another symptom. Difficulty in dealing with change is experienced. Exhaustion and fatigue, even on your days off, is another symptom. Lastly, a mentality that you have "checked out" or numb to situations is another symptom. ☐ Figure 7.6 describes the signs of physical and emotional exhaustion. ☐ Figure 7.7 describes signs of feelings of detachment and cynicism and ☐ Fig. 7.8 describes symptoms of a sense of ineffectiveness and a lack of accomplishment.

☐ Fig. 7.6 Signs of physical and emotional exhaustion

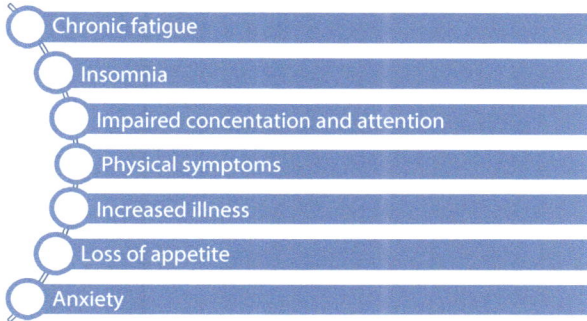

☐ Fig. 7.7 Signs of feelings of detachment and cynicism

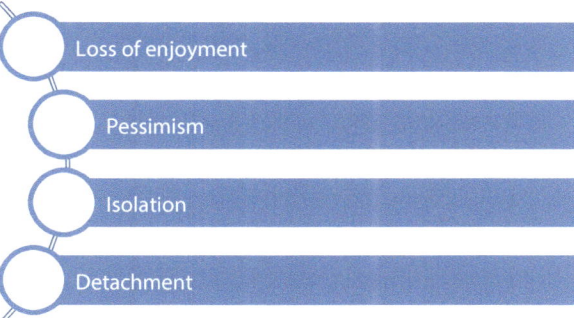

☐ Fig. 7.8 Symptoms of a sense of ineffectiveness and lack of accomplishment (Carter 2012)

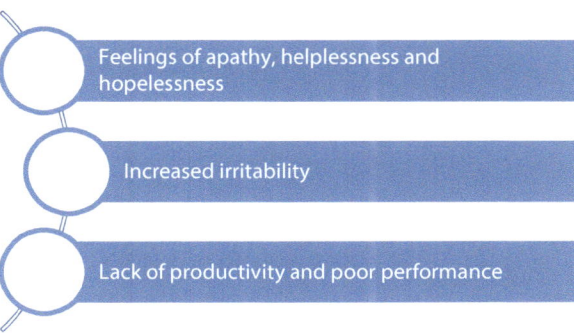

With each of these examples, early recognition and addressing signs of burnout is essential in the prevention of further burnout development. Prevention is also necessary, and the work environment may not be changed, but the registered nurses (RNs) can adjust whether the environment needs to be changed or if the RN needs to move to a different environment. Healthcare organizations typically offer counseling for registered nurses (RNs), which can include teaching stress management and self-care techniques. Adapting behaviors outside of work is important and can include keeping up professionally, separating home and work life, relaxing when off of work, eating healthy, exercising and getting adequate rest. Also, participating in non work related hobbies, meditation and journaling can all relieve stress.

Strategies

There are many strategies that can be used to develop professionally. Many online tools exist, some are evidence-based, some are not. The use of free tools should be used with caution as the information they provide is only a piece of information. If you do not agree with the findings, you should consider the further exploration of the topic to educate yourself best and ensure you put your best foot forward in building a successful nursing career.

1. Consider the following? Do they describe you?
   - Feelings of anxiety, irritability, fear, anger, moodiness. Thoughts of self-criticism, difficulty concentrating, making a decision, forgetful, mentally disorganizes, preoccupied with the future, repetitive thoughts, fear of failure
   - Behaviors such as crying, acting impulsively, nervous laughter, snap at a family and friends, teeth grinding, jaw clenching, smoking, alcohol or drug abuse
   - Physical sensations such as tight muscles, cold or sweaty hands, back or neck problems, difficulty sleeping, stomach aches, colds, infections, fatigue, rapid breathing, or pounding heart.
   - All of these coping methods may be detrimental to overall well-being.
2. This online quiz helps identify your level of kindness.
   How kind are you?
   Kindness Quiz: ▶ https://www.buildquizzes.com/QKU3TR
3. This online quiz helps identify your potential for developing burnout and your level of stress in the workplace.

   What is your stress level and potential for burnout? This online quiz helps evaluate the work environment. ▶ http://www.nursingleadership.org.uk/test5.php

   This online quiz helps assess the work environment and the presence of toxic work environments. How toxic is your work environment?

   ▶ https://www.nytimes.com/interactive/2015/06/21/opinion/sunday/incivility-at-work-quiz.html

   This quiz evaluates your understanding of workplace incivility: ▶ https://study.com/academy/practice/quiz-worksheet-workplace-incivility.html

❓ Activities

Activity 1: Building a successful nursing career requires ongoing work and the acceptance that you are on a lifelong journey of learning and professional development. Many activities are available to facilitate the journey. It is essential, to be honest with yourself, seek outside feedback when necessary, and strategize where you need to improve. This activity encourages you to explore your ability to contribute to your professional career. Is your tank on empty? Complete these worksheets to recognize your stress.

This worksheet evaluates what stress looks like for you and warning signs:
► https://www.mentalhealth.org.nz/assets/Working-Well/WS-tank-on-empty.pdf

How to reduce stress and burnout: ► https://www.airs.org/files/Difficult%20 Calls%20-%20Self%20Care%20Worksheet.pdf

❓ Activity 2

Consider the following scenarios and comments on incivility

Scenario #1:

You are a new graduate nurse practicing in a medical unit. There is a colleague that has been on the unit for seven years. One day after orientation, you hear her grumbling that "you need to pick up your pace; you are not pulling your weight." How might you handle this situation?

Comment

A direct approach is to acknowledge the offensive behavior head-on without offering excuses or opinions. You might say, "You criticize me a lot about my pace, and it distracts me from caring for my patients. I want you to stop making these comments so that I can focus on my patients." Confrontation can be challenging, but it often puts an end to the problem by directly addressing the offensive behavior.

Scenario #2:

You are sitting with several other colleagues catching-up on charting for the day. One of your colleagues starts gossiping and slamming another one of your colleagues. How might you handle this situation?

Comment

If someone is gossiping and slamming your colleague, do not join in or give approval by saying nothing. Have the courage to say, "I do not feel right talking about this behind his or her back. Have you talked with him or her?" It is important to hold each other accountable for our chosen behaviors.

Scenario #3:

You just walked out of a patient's room, when suddenly you hear a provider screaming and yelling at one of your colleagues. How might you handle this situation?

Comment

If you see someone being bullied, do not stand by quietly or pretend you do not see it. Unless each nurse names uncivil behavior when it occurs, it continues without any consequences. The behavior exhibited by the provider is unprofessional and should not be tolerated. One hospital uses a "code incivility" for each unit. When another person is bullying one of your colleagues, the rest of the nurses come and stand by the nurse being bullied, without saying a word. This action is usually enough to stop the behavior of the uncivil person and draws attention to their inappropriate behavior.

❓ Activity 3

Remember a time when you have been bullied by a peer or someone in leadership. Think about this situation and answer the questions below:

— How did the situation make you feel?
— Did you experience any of the listed feelings referred to in this chapter?
— How did you resolve the situation?
— Was it an assertive approach, or did you leave your position to get away from the incivility?
— How would you do things differently now?
— How do you manage stress reduction and taking care of yourself?

Vignettes

Vignette 1

The topics of civility and burnout in nursing often bring out anxiety among those who have been victims of incivility or experienced burnout. Below is a brief discussion of a registered nurse (RN) who experienced burnout and was unaware of how severe her burnout was.

I recently met with a registered nurse (RN). The meeting followed a request from her close colleagues, who stated she is not herself and not able to work effectively. When I begin my meeting, I intended to listen more, talk less. I wanted to find out what was going on. The meeting started with the registered nurse (RN) stating, "administration is putting too much on us and I cannot take it any longer!" I asked her to elaborate and give me some details so I could understand better. She went on to say, her colleagues were not helping her when she needed them, and they were letting her drown. She began to cry. I asked, "how can administration help with this problem?" She thought for a minute, grabbed another Kleenex then stated, "well, I guess I do not really accept their help, I want to do it myself. I need to do it myself to ensure it is done right." She went on to say that she is just tired, exhausted. I asked her when was the last time she took a day off for herself. She said she couldn't do that; she has too much responsibility outside of work as she is caring for her mother, who is ill. I stopped, thought to myself, this registered nurse (RN) is the picture of burnout….

We then turned the conversation to her and her self-care. We eventually agreed she would take some time off for herself then meet back in a couple of weeks. I saw her a couple of weeks later, she was not smiling, but she said the time was helpful and she felt she was not better but was going in the right direction…she underestimated how much her burnout impacted those around her and underestimated how little time she was giving to herself.

Vignette 2

How do you handle stress in your nursing job?

At the moment, I don't tend to feel the stress. I'm too intent on providing care for the patient and offering support to the doctors and team around me. Later, though, sometimes it hits me. My strategy is to go for a walk and listen to music.

Vignette 3

How do you handle working with a rude physician?

Everyone has bad days. If the rudeness is a one-time occurrence, I will let it go. If something significant happens, or if it's repeated, I'd reach out to my supervisor. My concern would be that perhaps the doctor was rude not because of a bad day, but because of dissatisfaction with my work.

Vignette 4

What is the best part of being a nurse?

As a maternity nurse, I'm there for the moment when people's family grows. It's powerful and awe-inspiring to witness. And I'm so happy to be able to reassure and help women in this big moment, especially first-time moms.

Vignette 5

How do you handle patients who complain of constant pain?

I would listen sympathetically to the patient's complaint and reassure him that his concerns were being heard and that we were doing everything possible to help. If it seemed warranted, I'd confer with the attending doctor to make sure that the patient's pain was being managed in the most effective way.

References

American Nurses Association (ANA) (2015) Incivility, bullying, and workplace violence. https://www.nursingworld.org/~49baac/globalassets/practiceandpolicy/nursing-excellence/official-policy-statements/ana-wpv-position-statement-2015.pdf

Carter SB (2012) Where do you fall on the burnout continuum? Psychol Today. https://www.psychologytoday.com/us/blog/high-octane-women/201205/where-do-you-fall-the-burnout-continuum

Clark CM (2010) Why civility matters. STTI. https://www.reflectionsonnursingleadership.org/features/more-features/Vol36_1_why-civility-matters

Clark CM (2013) Creating and sustaining civility in nursing education. Sigma Theta Tau, Indianapolis

Clark CM (2020) Conceptual model to foster civility in nursing education. https://www.boisestate.edu/research-ott/civility-matters-3/conceptual-models/conceptual-model-to-foster-civility-in-nursing-education/#:~:text=Conceptual%20Model%20to%20Foster%20Civility%20in%20Nursing%20Education.,high%20levels%20of%20faculty%20and%20student%20stress%20intersect

Compson J (2015) The CARE heuristic for addressing burnout in nurses. J Nurs Educ Pract 5(7):63–74. http://www.sciedu.ca/journal/index.php/jnep/article/view/6473

Kahl CS (2019) Making the invisible visible: capturing the multidimensional value of volunteerism to nonprofit organizations. Dissertations 139. https://digital.sandiego.edu/dissertations/139

Tillman C (2020) Incivility in nursing. http://otb.smsu.edu/annotated-works1/nursing-scholarly-annotated-Incivility%20in%20Nursing.html

University of California, Berkeley (2009) Social scientists build a case for 'survival of the kindest'. ScienceDaily, 9 Dec 2009. www.sciencedaily.com/releases/2009/12/091208155309.htm.

Waddill-Goad S (2016) Nurse burnout: overcoming stress in nursing. Nursing Knowledge.

Watson J (2011) Human caring science: a theory of nursing, 2nd edn. Jones and Bartlett Learning, Burlington

Wei H, Watson J (2019) Healthcare interprofessional team members' perspectives on human caring: a directed content analysis study. Int J Nurs Sci 6:17–23

Ensuring Continued Professional Growth

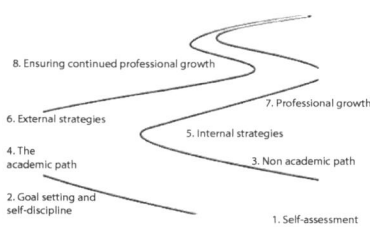

Contents

© Springer Nature Switzerland AG 2020
J. M. Manning, *The Path to Building a Successful Nursing Career*,
https://doi.org/10.1007/978-3-030-50023-8_8

Choose a job you love, and you will never have to work a day in your life. —Unknown author

Find out what you like doing best and get someone to pay you for doing it. —Katharine Whitehorn

I think one's feelings waste themselves in words; they ought all to be distilled into actions which bring results. —Florence Nightingale

8.1 Leadership Development

» Great leaders don't set out to be a leader; they set out to make a difference. It is never about the role, always about the goal. —Lisa Haisha

» Leadership is lifting a person's vision to higher sights, the raising of a persons performance to a higher standard. —Peter Drucker

8.1.1 What Is Leadership?

Peter Northouse defines leadership as "a process whereby an individual influences a group of individuals to achieve a common goal." Through this definition, it is clear that leadership is not a behavior or a trait. A job title does not make you a leader. Influence on others defines a leader.

8.1.2 Transformational Leadership

A political sociologist, James MacGregor Burns popularized the concept of transformational leadership in the late 1970s. According to Burns, transformational leaders are committed to a collective good through several key factors: idealized influence, inspirational motivation, intellectual stimulation, and individualized concern (◘ Fig. 8.1).

Idealized influence refers to the charisma leaders demonstrate, which results in followers supporting an established vision. Inspirational motivation is the use of com-

◘ **Fig. 8.1** Transformational leadership factors (Northouse 2020)

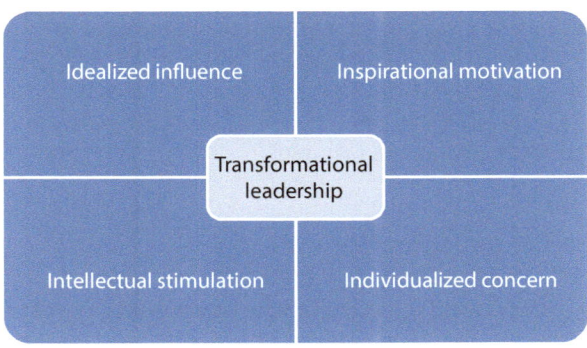

munication by the transformational leader to encourage others and inspire action. Intellectual stimulation fosters the use of innovation, thinking, and the challenging of assumptions by followers. Individualized concerns are the focus on the common good and demonstration of caring and concern for followers by the transformational leader.

8.1.3 Leadership Development Principles

Leadership development refers to activities that improve skills, abilities, and leader confidence. There are many leadership development programs for purchase by consumers—each of these programs shares some similarities one can adopt with diligence and commitment. For example, leadership coaches can be hired. Keep in mind success depends on support from mentors, your style, and acceptance to learn and expand your knowledge.

8.1.4 Self-Assessment

In ► Chap. 1, self-awareness was described. Effective leaders are self-aware. Understanding oneself helps with building a purpose, authenticity, trust, openness, and strong character. Our self-awareness helps explain our success and failures and helps to identify gaps in skills where additional work is needed. Those who are self-aware can make decisions to improve effectiveness. The self-awareness journey is an ongoing process and should be consistently reflected upon.

Remember, in leadership development, one size doesn't fit all. Be prepared for life-long learning. One must understand there will be learning, knowledge built and development. Awareness will provide insight. One should pursue the formal and informal approach. Leadership development must include self-assessment and self-reflection.

Leaders must be aware of how they are perceived by others. Effective leaders do not assume others understand your reasoning. Leaders must be transparent in their communication. They must also understand their weaknesses and work to overcome flaws in their skills.

8.1.5 Leadership Mindset

Leaders must appreciate the role of supporting, driving, guiding, and influencing others. How leaders respond to situations must be understood to ensure the leader is bringing out the best in followers. Leaders should develop a vision that sets the direction for success. A strong sense of purpose is essential for others to understand and become inspired.

8.1.6 Leading Others

Leaders need to understand accountability, outcomes, and effectiveness. They must manage the conditions which drive the performance of individuals and teams.

Supporting team goals, processes, and the leader must provide goal achievement of others.

Leaders should have excellent people skills. These should include the ability to observe others, communicate effectively, motivate others, and adapt. Leaders should genuinely connect with others. This is necessary for the development of trust and, ultimately, a productive work environment.

8.1.7 Maximize Leadership Potential

Leaders must understand their style of leadership and how it intersects with the goals of the organization. Leaders must know how to motivate the individual talents of followers and teams. Understanding your own values and internal motivators are essential in maximizing leadership potential. A leader must be decisive and make sound judgments. Leaders should know when a quick decision is needed and must be able to make a firm decision (► Case Example 8.1).

8.1.8 Networking

A leader must understand how to influence through coaching and feedback delivery. Leveraging resources are necessary for expansion and development. Leaders must manage stress effectively. There should be a clear understanding of the context of leadership in the organization. The leader must learn what leadership is and the impression of an effective leader in organizations. Development through mentoring and coaching can be useful.

Leaders must be able to collaborate and understand all great ideas do not come from only the leader. Collaboration is key to success and creating an environment where ideas can be shared benefits the organization.

Case Example 8.1 Tips for Leadership Success

1. Work with those you respect and learn from them
2. For you (and those you lead), make family a priority. If you focus on your family, your work will be a success
3. Do not burn bridges
4. Talk less and listen more
5. Seek a mentor you can confide in and seek guidance from them
6. Be open to new ideas, don't draw lines in the sand; ask how we can step across the lines
7. Read and learn something new every day
8. Prepare. Be the person in the room who is prepared, speak up when necessary and listen carefully
9. Start and advance the conversation. Do not avoid and end conversations
10. Do not lose your sense of humor
11. Be enthusiastic

8.1.9 Leading in the Nursing Profession

Nurses are commonly encouraged to pursue leadership roles because of a strong history of clinical expertise. Staff nurses use leadership skills when transitioning to a new leadership role such as a charge nurse, nurse manager, etc. Some of the hallmark skills of a nurse leader in a formal leadership role include authenticity, communication, relationship building, collaboration, accountability, transparency, accessibility, transparency, and trust.

Formal nurse leadership roles, such as the nurse manager, have become increasingly complex, and the accountability and responsibilities are many. These include responsibility for department operations, human resource outcomes, department quality, etc. The fiscal and economic outcomes the formal nurse leader face may include oversight of multiple nursing units and large numbers of direct reports. Accountability shifts to a 24/7 expectation and expectations for ensuring staffing; patient care outcomes are ongoing top priorities. Formal nurse leaders have one often most challenging jobs in the organizational structure of healthcare.

8

8.1.10 The Path to Leading in the Nursing Profession

Unfortunately, formal nurse leaders learn their new role on the job and lack formal leadership training and formal mentors. Their hours are more than 40 hours per week and positive feedback is not always ongoing from upper-level administration and direct reports. They are often faced with work–life balance challenges and the need for more autonomy, empowerment, and recognition in their role in health care organizations.

Development in the role could be enhanced through a leadership development program. The American Nurses Association and the American Organization of Nurse Leaders offer training to assist in leadership development. The training can be virtual via computer-based learning modules and webinars or in-person workshops, conferences, and structured programs. Fellowship programs exist which are held for up to a year and include didactic education, networking, mentorship, and reflective learning strategies.

Organizations with resources to support the onboarding of a formal nurse leader can meet many of the new leader's needs. Smaller organizations may not have as many resources. Upper administration can facilitate the leader's development. Programs can improve problem-solving, creativity, networking, and support. Through these programs, the formal nurse leaders can implement shared decision-making principles.

A key to success for the formal nurse leader should include skills in their ability to recruit, engage, and retain nursing staff. Their confidence and skills can be enhanced. These outcomes are described in the Future of Nursing report issued by the Institute of Medicine (2010), where nurses are challenged to practice nursing to the full extent of their education and training as well as to choose higher levels of education to support the role they are working in. The success of a formal nurse leader requires skills and competency development that are unique to the role. Unfortunately, organizations do not have formal programs available, and the nurse leader must seek these development opportunities on their own.

8.1.11 American Organization for Nursing Leadership: Leader Competencies

The AONL's mission is to shape healthcare through innovative and expert leadership. Core competencies for nurse leaders are described based on a variety of settings and levels of responsibilities. They include nurse executive competencies, system nurse executive competencies, post-acute care competencies, nurse manager competencies, nurse executive competencies: population health, and nurse leader skill assessments.

The nurse manager competencies include a framework that encompasses several domains: the science, the leader within, and the art of the nurse manager (◘ Fig. 8.2 and ◘ Table 8.1).

◘ **Fig. 8.2** The American Organization for Nursing Leadership Nurse Manager Competencies. (AONL Nurse Manager competencies. Retrieved from: ▸ https://www.aonl.org/system/files/media/file/2019/04/nurse-manager-competencies.pdf)

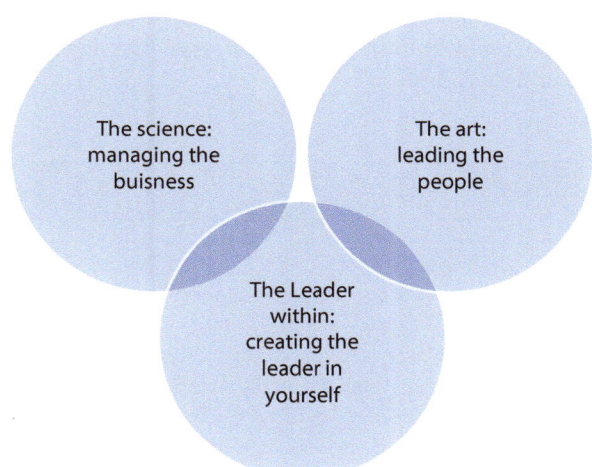

◘ **Table 8.1** American Organization for Nursing Leadership Nurse Manager Competency Domain Descriptions

The Science domain	Financial management Human resources management Performance improvement Foundational thinking skills Technology skills Strategic management Clinical practice knowledge
The Leader within domain	*Personal and professional accountability* *Career planning* *Personal journey disciplines* *Optimizing the leader within*
The Art domain	*Human resource leadership skills* *Relationship management* *Influencing behaviors* *Diversity* *Shared decision-making*

The science domain includes the skills and competencies related to fiscal management, human resources management, performance improvement, foundational thinking skills, technology skills, strategic management, and clinical practice knowledge. The Leader Within domain addresses the creation of the leader within oneself and includes personal and professional accountability, career planning, individual journey disciplines, and optimizing the leader within. The Art domain consists of the leading of people through human resource leadership skills, relationship management, influencing behaviors, diversity, and shared decision-making (◘ Table 8.1).

AONL describes reflective practice behaviors in leaders which include holding the truth, appreciation of ambiguity, diversity as a vehicle to wholeness, holding multiple perspectives without judgment, the discovery of potential, quest for adventure towards knowing, knowing something of life, nurturing the intellectual and emotional self, and keeping commitments to oneself (▶ Case Example 8.2).

8

> **Case Example 8.2 American Organization for Nursing Leadership Reflective Practice Behaviors within Leaders**
>
> 1. *Holding the truth*
>   The presence of integrity as a key value of leadership
> 2. *Appreciation of ambiguity*
>   Learning to function comfortably amid the ambiguity of our environments
> 3. *Diversity as a vehicle to wholeness*
>   The appreciation of diversity in all forms: race, gender, religion, sexual orientation, generational, the dissenting voice and differences of all kinds
> 4. *Holding multiple perspectives without judgement*
>   Creation and holding a space so that multiple perspectives are entertained before decisions are rendered
> 5. *Discovery of potential*
>   The ability to search for and find the potential in ourselves and in others
> 6. *Quest for adventure towards knowing*
>   Creating a constant state of learning for the self, as well as an organization
> 7. *Knowing something of life*
>   The use of reflective learning and translation of that learning to the work at hand
> 8. *Nurturing the intellectual and emotional self*
>   Constantly increasing one's knowledge of the world and the development of the emotional self
> 9. *Keeping commitments to oneself*
>   Creating the balance that regenerates and renews the spirit and body so that it can continue to grow
>   ▶ https://www.aonl.org/resources/nurse-leader-competencies

Nurse leaders maintain integrity by being honest with the staff. Through this honesty, trust is built by the leader in their role. The development of comfort in the role begins with an awareness of strengths and weaknesses. Self-awareness is essential in recognizing where the leader is acclimating quickly and where uneasiness is taking over. The appreciation of diversity in people and what they bring to the organization is essential. Most success comes from a variety of ideas that come from diverse groups in the organization, all contributing to a common goal. The ability to evaluate a situation from multiple angles and perspectives is vital in decision-making to ensure the leader is making the best possible decision. Comfort comes into play here as one cannot overthink to the point that the leader becomes indecisive.

Leadership potential is another critical area where the leader must explore their potential in not only themselves but in others. Identification of leadership potential is essential to ensure the leader is putting the right people in the right place at the right time. A constant thirst for knowledge is vital as there is a continuous learning curve in complex and dynamic healthcare environments. Translation of formal education into usable skills in the work environment is critical. Regular training programs are only as good as what the individual puts into practice. Leaders must continuously nurture their emotional selves. In the world of healthcare, where patient care outcomes and staff outcomes impact, people can take a toll on a leader, and developing one's emotional self is critical. Balance in regenerating and reenergizing oneself is essential in nursing leadership. The emotion and physical toll can be immense, and building self-care into daily life can ensure the leader does not burn out (Tomasko 2020; Leadership Development Model 2020; Oswald-Herold 2018).

8.2 Keeping Current

Staying up to date is an important skill when ensuring continued professional growth. The healthcare field has changed significantly in recent years. The internet and social media have transitioned to further development of decision support tools and patient management systems. There are several strategies one can use to stay up to date on topics relevant to the nursing profession.

8.2.1 Peer to Peer Interactions

Communicating and networking with colleges about new strategies and breakthroughs is a quick way to share information. Interacting with leaders in your field is great way to obtain information.

8.2.2 Healthcare Journals

Healthcare journals have been the traditional, primary method by which nurses receive information in their field. Complex data is disseminated to broad international audiences often through a peer-review process. Data that is published in rigorous peer-review journals can be viewed as quality research that is accurate and relevant. Top leaders often highlight their findings through journals. Also, expert opinions are offered to audiences regarding information as it relates to nursing practice.

8.2.3 Attend Conferences

Attending a conference is also a traditional method by which nurses stay up to date. Both large and small meetings provide an environment where experts can share information about the most recent breakthroughs, techniques, and research findings. The attendees are free from work and home distractions and can immerse themselves in a dedicated learning environment. In addition to the educational environment conferences offer, there is also a social environment where peers can network and interact about topics. They can focus on breaking data, clinical challenges, and future directions for the profession.

8

8.2.4 Decision Support Tools

The incorporation of decision support tools can include algorithms or guidelines which have been published for a specific issue. There are many benefits in using decision support tools such as they often follow the most up to date guidelines and research findings available. References are typically provided to show what sources were used to develop the tool. Tools can be updated as new information is published.

8.2.5 Continuous Learning

Every nurse should adopt a strategy of continuous learning. For many, professional development activities are a way to fulfill the ongoing learning needs of nurses. The benefit of professional development is that it filters through the immense amount of data available on a daily basis. An expert can interpret the updates and filter the information in a manner which is understandable for attendees. Multiple formats are available for learners such as face to face, webinar, interactive simulations, and learning management systems. Attendees should be selective in the developments they attend. They should be offered by an accredited institution. The information should be relevant to the learner and build upon their weaknesses.

8.2.6 Join an Organization

Join an organization which supports your area of interest. For example, a national nursing organization. These organizations can link you with a tremendous amount of resources. Use all of the resources available to you as a result of your membership. Many organizations offer professional development materials.

In addition to your area of interest, consider where you want to develop your expertise. For example, do you want to communicate better? Or become more organized? Or develop your leadership skills? Or your writing skills? Each of these skills are critical in further development. Some tools for development in these areas include:

For development of business skills:
- Harvard business review
- Harvard Business Schools Reading List: there are many books out there, this list will make sure you are making the most of your time in selecting some of the best.
- Forbes.com
- Ted.com: TED talks have some compelling presentations on business strategies, all for free. Eleven helpful resources for improving your business skills. Retrieved from: ▶ https://blog.hubspot.com/marketing/business-resources

For research summaries in nursing:
- National Institute of Nursing Research (NINR)
- Nursing Research
- Agency for Healthcare Research and Quality (AHRQ)
- National Database of Nursing Quality Indicators (NDNQI)
- PubMed
- National Councils for State Boards of Nursing (NCSBN)
- ANA Smart Brief

To improve your knowledge of your organization
- Your organizations annual report and strategic plan
- Join a committee outside of your department

For best practice:
- White papers
- National guidelines
- Periodic literature reviews

Keeping abreast of current events, even those in the nursing world can be a significant challenge. One must be strategic in managing knowledge and keeping current.

8.3 Ongoing Professional Development

Successful ongoing professional development must be be self-directed, driven by you. Not by your employer. The focus must be on learning from experience, reflective learning, and review. Mentors can help you set development goals and objectives. Learning should be formal and informal.

The cycle of ongoing professional development includes five main steps (◘ Fig. 8.3).

■ **Fig. 8.3**   The cycle of ongoing professional development

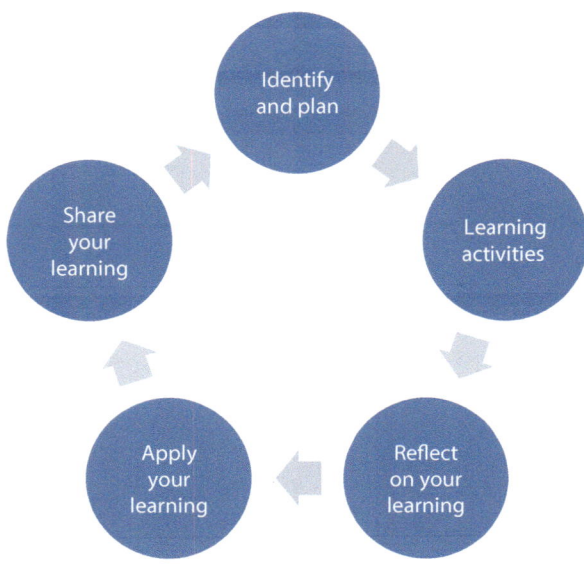

1. Identify your needs

Audit your skills. Obtain feedback from colleagues. Identify your interests and develop your knowledge.

2. Plan and carry out development activities

Formal training includes training courses. Usually, there is an external provider and an associated cost. There may be limitations to what you can pay, or your employer can supplement. Online resources may be cheaper, explore your options.

Informal learning can include side by side learning or video training. Also, coaching or reading on the subject.

Professional development is essential and potentially expensive. Be imaginative in your approach and seek developments that work for you.

3. Reflect on your learning

Reflect on what you have learned. Learning doesn't occur and emerges from activities alone. It is how you incorporate your learning into your day to day activities. Following the activity, document what you found useful and not useful. Also, include what you have learned.

4. Apply your learning

The application of your learning can be clumsy at first. It includes first identifying what you didn't know, and now you know it. Transitioning that knowledge to your competency is essential, and if consistently applied, it becomes part of your skillset.

5. Share your learning with others

Teaching others is the next step in this cycle. Whether through mentorship or in a formal setting. Demonstrate your new skills. Keep an ongoing note of your needs and goals. Regularly assess your progress in achieving them.

This process is a cycle; it is ongoing. It is a journey, not a destination.

» Whatever you do, do it well. —Walt Disney

Strategies

Complete these free online quizzes:

Are you a leader? ► https://psychologia.co/leadership-test/

What is my leadership style? ► https://www.mindtools.com/pages/article/leadership-style-quiz.htm

Develop your leadership skills with this worksheet: ► https://www.institutelm.com/learning/worksheets.html

Activity

Some activities for ongoing professional development include:

► https://managementhelp.org/leadership/development/index.htm

1. Keep a note of your needs and goals. Visit these goals on a regular basis, either yearly or biannually.
2. Record what you have learned in trainings.
3. Shadow others.
4. Secure mentors.
5. When you encounter a resource, you want to know more about, make a note, and work on it when you visit your goals.
6. When you are involved in critical events, make notes of the mistakes you make and work on those weaknesses.

Vignettes

Vignette 1

I recently asked a fellow registered nurse (RN) leader; how do you stay on top of everything? There is so much information out there? She said she does the following:

1. Acknowledges that every learning opportunity she seeks will not be the most beneficial, but if she doesn't try, she will never know.
2. She takes advantage of summaries from the organizations she subscribes to. For example, the ANA offers a weekly SmartBrief which summarizes the literature into a newsletter format she can quickly read.
3. She uses Twitter to create her unique news, she follows organizations she wants ongoing updates from and reviews twitter like a newspaper. Reads the headlines, then reads further if she wants to know more information.

4. She shares pertinent information with her colleagues; she forwards information to those she leads so they have the most up to date information.
5. Lastly, she acknowledges she can't know it all and listens to others and searches for information every day so she can do the best job possible with the information she has.

Vignette 2
An interview with the ANA president, Ernest Grant
   This interview details how Dr. Grant became a nurse. His specialized area of interest. What he loves about nursing. The challenges he sees for nursing and where he wants the ANA to go in the future (Skidmore 2018; Thew 2018; HRZone 2020).

References

HRZone (2020) What is leadership development? https://www.hrzone.com/hr-glossary/what-is-leadership-development
Institute of Medicine. (2010). The future of nursing: Leading change, advancing health. Retrieved from http://books.nap.edu/openbook.php?record_id=12956&page=R1
Leadership Development Model (2020). http://www.nwlink.com/~donclark/leadership/development/leadership_development_model.html
Northouse (2020) Leadership theory and practice. SAGE Publications, New York
Oswald-Herold C (2018) A review of literature and taxonomy of leadership development programs. https://www.501commons.org/learn/research/foundational-emerging-models-of-leadership-development
Skidmore K (2018) 17 Elements to include in leadership development programs. https://www.flashpointleadership.com/blog/guide-to-leadership-development-by-leader-level
Thew J (2018) Q & A with the first man elected as American nurses association president. Health Leaders. https://www.healthleadersmedia.com/nursing/qa-first-man-elected-american-nurses-association-president
Tomasko R (2020) Seven models of leadership development. http://www.roberttomasko.com/Consult.7ModelsLead.html

Professionalism

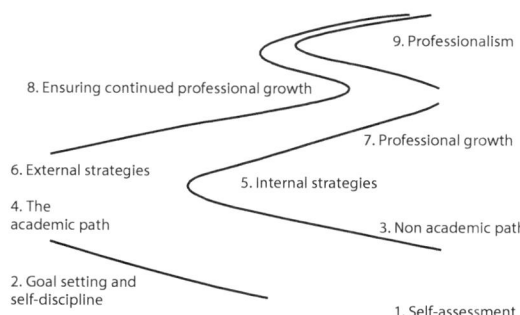

Contents

© Springer Nature Switzerland AG 2020
J. M. Manning, *The Path to Building a Successful Nursing Career*,
https://doi.org/10.1007/978-3-030-50023-8_9

"Professional is not a label you give yourself....

– it is a description you hope others will apply to you" —David Maister

9.1 Professional Behavior

Professional behavior is a form of etiquette in the workplace that is primarily linked to respectful and courteous conduct. The meaning of "professional" has been a topic among scholars for nearly 100 years. There is a general consensus that a profession is an occupational group of people with a similar set of attitudes and behaviors (Black 2016). In 2017, Abraham Flexner published professional criteria that reformed medical education in the early 1900s. According to Flexner, a profession includes:

- An intellectual accompanied by a high degree of individual responsibility.
- Based on a body of knowledge that can be learned and developed as well as refined with research.
- Practical and theoretical.
- Can be taught through specialized professional education programs.
- Practitioners are motivated by altruism and are responsive to public interests.

In the 1980s, a nurse scholar Lucie Kelly compiled eight characteristics of a profession that remain embodied by nursing.

1. A service provided that is vital to humanity and society.
2. A special body of knowledge that is developed through research.
3. The service includes intellectual activities and individual responsibility.
4. Practitioners are educated in higher learning institutions.
5. Practitioners are somewhat independent and control their own policies and activities.
6. Practitioners are motivated by service and consider their work important.
7. A code of ethics guides decisions.
8. An organization encourages and supports high standards of practice.

9.1.1 Service Provided Is Vital to Humanity and the Welfare of Society

One of the most common reasons a person wants to become a nurse is to "help people." Nursing provides an essential service to people and society. Nurses provide care to patients through caring service.

9.1.2 A Unique Body of Knowledge That Is Developed Through Research

Nursing has a broad collection of knowledge, with scholars and researchers expanding the science of nursing knowledge every day. Nursing relies on theory and research to support best practices.

9.1.3 **The Service Includes Intellectual Activities, Individual Responsibility**

Nursing requires critical and creative thinking. Nursing has a unique approach to practice, called the nursing process. The nursing process is a modified scientific method and functions as a guide to patient centered care. The steps in the nursing process include assessment, nursing diagnosis, planning, implementation and evaluation (■ Fig. 9.1). Individual accountability is the hallmark of nursing practice. The ANA code of ethics for nursing states a nurse is "responsible and accountable for individual nursing practice and determines the appropriate delegation of tasks consistent with the nurse's obligation to provide optimum patient care."

9.1.4 **Practitioners Are Educated in Higher Learning Institutions**

The first nursing program began in 1909 at the University of Minnesota. In 1965, the ANA published a position paper stating that all nursing education should occur in higher education institutions. The long-held debate regarding entry-level into practice remains. Currently, Associate Degree Nursing Programs remain the

9

■ **Fig. 9.1**   Nursing process

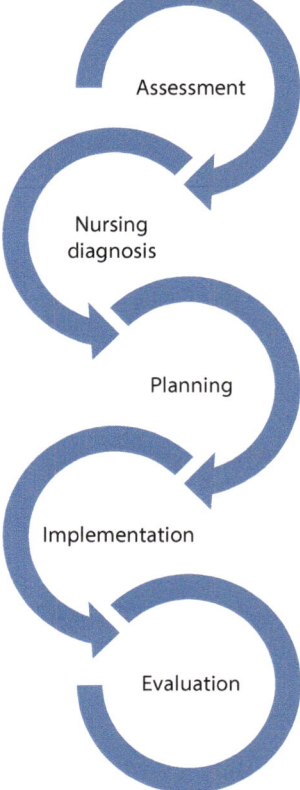

primary source of entry-level registered nurses. The number of Diploma programs and BSN programs has decreased over the past 30 years. The number of Masters and Doctoral programs continues to increase.

9.1.5 Practitioners Are Somewhat Independent and Control Their Policies and Activities

Nursing boards license nurses. Most nurses are employed in settings where their actions are interdependent, where physician orders, APRN orders, and physician orders are carried out by RNs. Nurses face many practice constraints in performing to the full scope of their training. Several groups outside of nursing have attempted to control nursing practice. They include medicine, and health service administration professional bodies. The interests of these bodies are expressed through state and federal lobbying efforts, which aim to influence legislation and, ultimately, nursing practice scope and autonomy.

9.1.6 Practitioners Are Motivated by Service and Consider Their Work Important

Nurses are dedicated to the service of others. This service is not always the defining identity of many nurses. Nursing is intertwined with economic factors, which include the need to charge reasonable fees for services rendered. Higher compensation and improved working conditions have been requested for many years. Nurses must be responsible and a voice for their own financial needs.

In nursing careers, professional behavior is essential. Registered nurse (RN) need to provide high-quality care in complex healthcare environments. The American Nurses Association (ANA) describes standards of excellence to promote the high standards of ethics, effectiveness, and accountability in nursing practice. The standards of excellence include professional standards that elevate the nursing profession by defining the values and priorities for registered nurses nationwide. These professional standards support the objective evaluation of nursing excellence and include the code of ethics for nurses, ANA nursing standards, ANA position statements, and ANA principles of nursing practice. The code of ethics defines how nurses should deliver care in an ethical manner. The nursing standards, or scope and standards of practice, describe the art and science of nursing practice. The position statements address hot topic areas that explain, justify, or recommend a course of action in a specific area. The principles for nursing practice address cutting edge topics such as staffing, delegation, and social media and provide practical information for professional nursing practice.

Nine characteristics have been identified to describe professionalism (◨ Fig. 9.2). They include appearance, demeanor, reliable, organized, ethical, poised, etiquette (verbal and written), accountable, and professional boundaries.

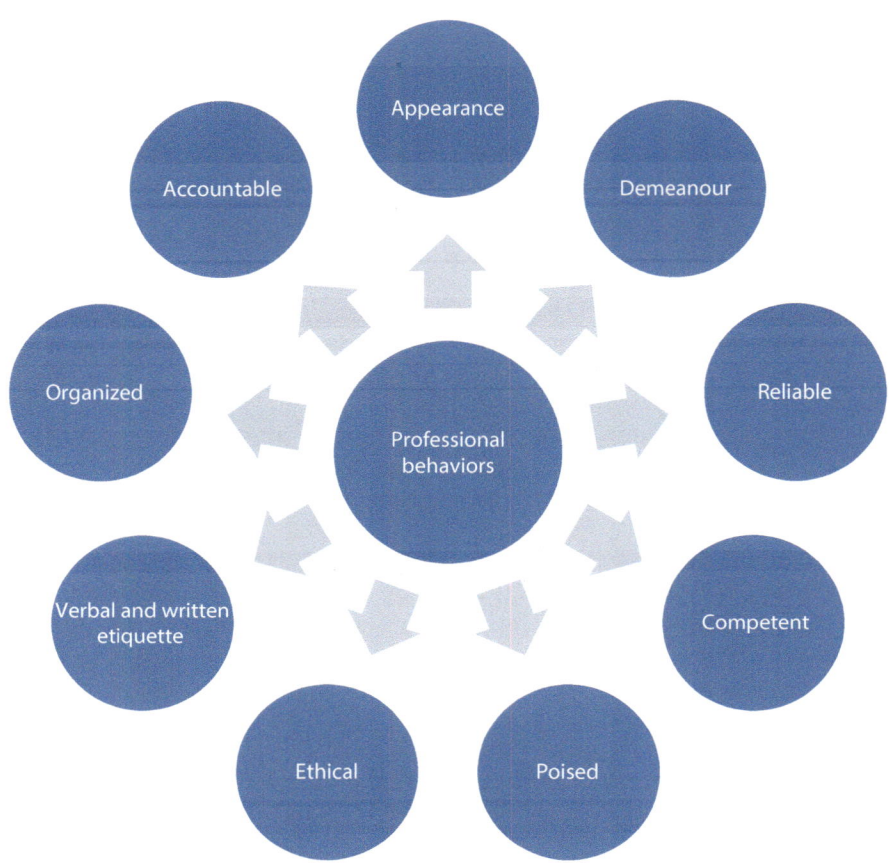

☐ **Fig. 9.2**   Professional behaviors

9.1.7 **Appearance**

A professional is neat and clean in appearance. They meet or exceed organizational dress code requirements. They are especially aware of their appearance when meeting with those outside of the organization (e.g., clients or applicants).

A professional registered nurse (RN) appearance influences patient care. How a registered nurse (RN) dresses conveys professionalism and confidence to patients. Historically how registered nurses (RNs) dressed was strictly enforced. Today, the "image of nursing" is a much-debated topic. In a clinical setting, the best approach is simple and functional with plain colors, clean and neat with a prominent display of "RN" is a good guideline to follow.

9.1.8 Demeanor

A professional's behavior should be confident, polite, and well-spoken in all inter-actions. Even when identified as an expert, the way a professional treats others is critical. A professional is warm and friendly but not too friendly. For example, the use of "sweetie" is not appropriate. Similar to above, a licensed (RN)'s demeanor should include clear communication, consistency, and respect. Registered nurses (RNs) always heal the sick, nurture the wounded, put patients first, provide holistic care, and educate the new professional registered nurses (RNs) in training.

A nurse's demeanor should align with the practice standards and broader goals of their organizations. A nurse should be willing to be flexible and make compro-mises for the greater good when navigating professional challenges (Bostain 2020).

9.1.9 Reliable

A professional is reliable and can be counted on to complete the job at hand. Prompt response to others and following through on promised work is essential. Professionals meet expectations through effective communication. Clarification is sought to ensure everyone is on the same page without surprises. Professional reg-istered nurses (RNs) play a key role in improving the reliability of healthcare. Through their reliable work, they can shape and advance quality and safety pro-cesses (Hancock 2020).

9.1.10 Organized

A professional is organized and can find what is needed. Their work area is neat, and they bring what is needed for a presentation or appointment. Professional registered nurses (RNs) must approach care delivery in an organized manner with a key focus on prioritization and delegation of responsibilities to others.

9.1.11 Competent

A professional seeks to become an expert in their field to set themselves apart from others. Professional development is described further in ▶ Chap. 8. Professional registered nurses (RNs) must demonstrate competence, which is often the founda-tion for nursing education curricula. Competency in risk management, basic responsibilities, care coordination, professional development, improvement of nursing quality, and health promotion are some of the key areas where a professional registered nurse (RN) must demonstrate competency (Fukada 2018; Sortedahl et al. 2017).

9.1.12 Ethical

A professional adheres to a strict code of ethics, even unwritten rules. A nurse should always exhibit ethical behavior, without exception. A licensed registered nurse (RN) adheres to a strict code of ethics, which is described by the American registered nurses (RNs) association. Nine provisions are described and address the ethical values, obligations, and duties of everyone entering the nursing profession. Ethical standards in nursing are not negotiable, and a registered nurse (RN) must express their understanding of nursing's commitment to society.

Nurses should be honest and demonstrate integrity. They should always aspire to high levels of personal and professional conduct (▶ https://www.nursingworld. org/practice-policy/nursing-excellence/ethics/).

9.1.13 Poised

A professional registered nurse (RN) must maintain poise, as described previously for all professionals. The impact on transforming practice is at stake. A professional maintains composure at all times, especially in stressful situations. The ability to keep calm and structured during challenging circumstances is essential while staying on task and moving forward clearly and directly. Persons with high Emotional Intelligence (described in ▶ Chap. 1) avoid losing their cool in tense situations. They also do not air their emotional baggage which can result in loss of integrity, credibility, and reputation (▶ https://www.ncbi.nlm.nih.gov/books/NBK209871/).

9

9.1.14 Etiquette in Verbal Communication and Written Correspondence

» The single biggest problem in communication is the ILLUSION that it has taken place. —George Bernard Shaw

» What you do speaks so loudly, I can't hear what you say! —Ralph Waldo Emerson

Nurses must possess high-level communication skills. Through skilled communication, they can provide care by listening to others, provide information, advise patients in a manner which is clear and understandable. Nurses can make well-informed decisions that are in the best interest of the patient. Their skills must demonstrate etiquette in verbal and written correspondence (■ Fig. 9.3).

9.1.14.1 Verbal Communication

Registered nurses (RNs) must learn essential communication skills and must understand the message they send through their communication. Communication is verbal and nonverbal. Nonverbal includes eye contact, voice tone, body language, posture, and the use of a smile. Verbal communication includes active listening, which is the form of listening with the goal of understanding. Demonstration of a level of interest to build trust with patients and colleagues. The ability to

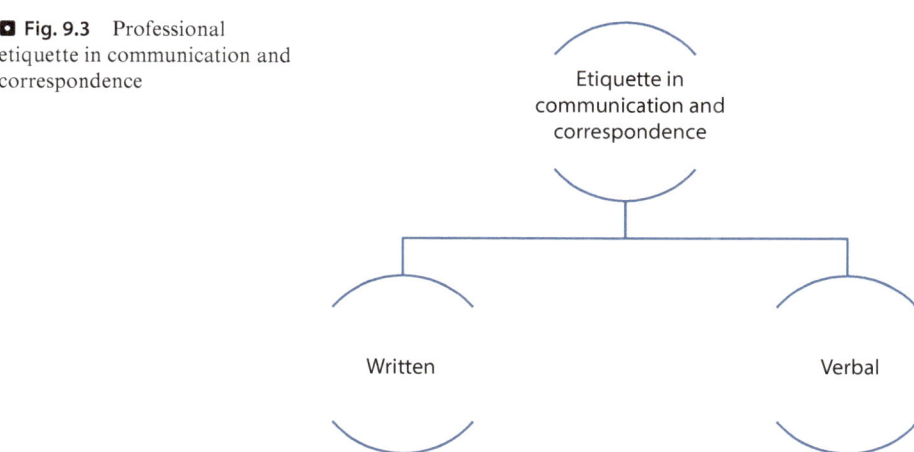

inspire trust by listening to complaints and maintaining confidentiality. The ability to show compassion by respecting the dignity of others. Cultural awareness is essential with respect to other cultural practices. Communication through patient education is essential with the ability to ensure self-care and use of the teach-back model. The ability to present to others based on the audience's level of understanding is an essential skill. Professional registered nurses (RNs) must be clear in their communication with an awareness of their tone.

Public speaking is rarely a favorite activity for many and often instills fear in some. Unfortunately, it is hard to be a spokesperson for an organization without engaging in some public speaking. Through speaking, you establish authority and credibility in a group. There are many strategies to improve speaking skills. Unfortunately, the only way to improve this skill is actually to do it. Start small, speak at a staff meeting, or provide an in-service to a couple of people. Then increase the size of the group. Work on your poise and self-confidence to ensure your ideas are heard.

9.1.14.2 Written Correspondence

Written communication must be easy to understand with correct grammar and spelling. The use of medical jargon must be used only when appropriate. Verbal *Correspondence*: Professional identity by stating their full name, company, and title in phone conversations. They do not dominate conversations and actively listen to others. Written *Correspondence*: Professionals keep written information brief and to the point. The tone is always polite and formal. Avoid being overly polite. Written correspondence is a paper trail and record of transactions. Care should always be taken when writing statements. Use correct spelling and grammar. Never use ALL CAPITALS, regardless of the level of frustration you are experiencing.

Writing letters is a powerful tool to support others while they increase organizational visibility. If someone has done something great, write them a thank-you note. This provides praise and ensures cooperation in the future. Include their supervisor as a powerful message and secondary benefit to the person you are thanking. This strategy is not self-serving; it is essential that we support each other in organizations.

The result is strengthening the organization. In the same light, if you receive a letter of support, keep it or ask if the person will put it in writing. The written form validates your abilities and can be used when applying for a job or promotion.

9.1.15 Accountable

Professionals are accountable for their actions. When they make a mistake, they own it and try to fix the error. They do not blame others. They compromise when working on resolving issues. They use opportunities to gain the respect of others and handle situations. (▶ https://www.linkedin.com/pulse/10-characteristics-professionalism-greg).

In addition to these professional behaviors, registered nurses (RNs) must expect and *anticipate change*. The healthcare environment is dynamic, and often change occurs with little to no notice. Maintaining composure and clear thinking is essential during the transition. Registered nurses (RNs) must also *learn from their failures*. They must be able to reflect on past behaviors, constructively criticize, and improve. This skill is essential as patient care is different every day, and no two patients are alike. Lastly, the registered nurses (RNs) must *manage conflict* with skill and compassion. Patients are typically experiencing some of the most challenging times of their lives, and their response is not always positive leading to stressful situations. Registered nurses (RNs) must learn to master conflict resolution to a leader in healthcare environments. These professional behaviors are essential for development in registered nurses (RNs) as they transition through their careers (▶ Case Example 9.1).

Case Example 9.1 Professional Behaviors

Change
Expect change
How to manage change
How to respond to resistance to change
How to propose solutions
Willingness to give recommendations
Understand change theory
How to apply change theory to appropriate situations
▶ https://journals.lww.com/neponline/FullText/2017/11000/Essential_Professional_Behaviors_of_Nursing.3.aspx

---

9.1.16 Professional Boundaries

Professional registered nurses (RNs) must understand and apply concepts of professional boundaries. The repeated emphasis on nursing as the most widely respected and trusted profession is reflected by the special relationships between registered nurses (RNs) and those under their care. All patients expect registered nurses (RNs) to act in their best interest, advocate for them, and respect the patient dignity. Professional boundaries are the intimate space between the power of a registered nurse (RN) and a patient's vulnerability. Registered nurses (RNs) must respect this power and demonstrate a patient-centered relationship.

Boundaries are violated when confusion between the registered nurse (RN) and the patient occurs. Violations include excessive personal disclosure, secrecy, or reversal of registered nurse (RN)/patient roles. When boundaries are crossed, even when unintended, the registered nurse (RN) must attempt to re-establish boundaries. A repeat of the boundary crossing must not occur. Boundaries are violated when there is confusion between the patient and registered nurse (RN) needs.

With social media, new types of boundary crossing, and violations are occurring. Registered nurses (RNs) are challenged with being aware of boundary crossing and violations on the internet. They must be cognizant of feelings and behaviors. They must observe the behavior of other professionals. They must act in the best interest of the patient, always (▶ https://www.ncsbn.org/professional-boundaries. htm). ◘ Figure 9.4 describes some "red flag" behaviors which may indicate professional boundary issues.

◘ **Fig. 9.4**   Red flag behaviors
(▶ https://www.ncsbn.org/
ProfessionalBoundaries_
Complete.pdf)

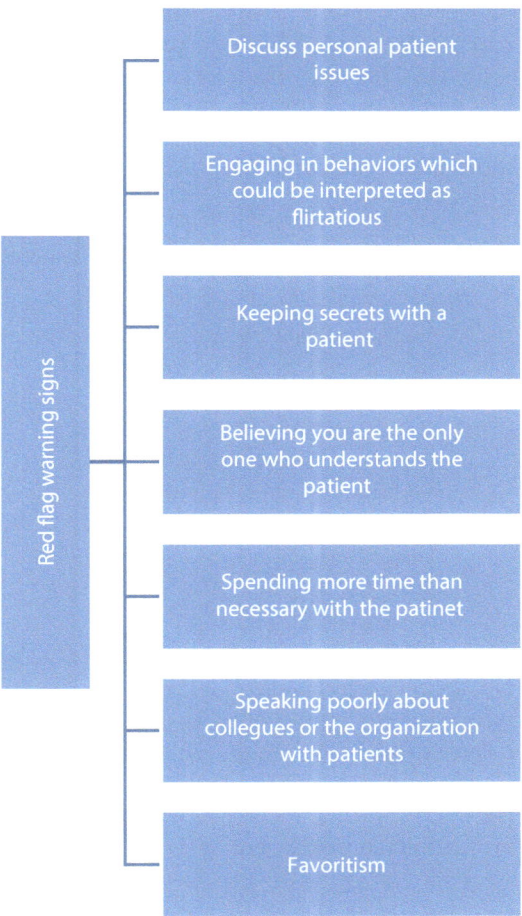

Red flag warning signs

- Discuss personal patient issues
- Engaging in behaviors which could be interpreted as flirtatious
- Keeping secrets with a patient
- Believing you are the only one who understands the patient
- Spending more time than necessary with the patinet
- Speaking poorly about collegues or the organization with patients
- Favoritism

9.2 **Ethics**

The study of ethics has been a focus for scholars for many years. Ethics is a branch of philosophy defined as the study of ideal human behavior and ideal ways of being (Black 2016). The meanings of ethical concepts aim to understand, analyze, and distinguish good and bad, right and wrong along a continuum. Decisions regarding ethics are made through the applied use of ethical theories and ethical codes of conduct. Bioethics is a domain of ethics that focuses on healthcare moral issues. Callahan (2002) defined bioethics as "an intersection of ethic and life sciences."

9.2.1 **Nursing Ethics**

Nursing ethics can be viewed as a subcategory of bioethics. Understanding ethical concepts is essential to prepare nurses to work through practice-based situations where ethical implications occur. Ethics are fundamental to nursing practice. Nurses encounter everyday situations where ethics play a role such as in the case of making decisions about how to prioritize and allocate time and resources, how to share information with patients, how to work with challenges among colleagues, how to resolve problems, and when there are conflicts among institutional policies and patient care delivery. ▶ Case Example 9.2 describes strategies to manage through ethical conflicts.

9

Case Example 9.2 Ethical Conflict Management

Strategies to Manage Through Ethical Conflicts:
  Understand why conflict occurs
  Learn conflict resolution techniques
  Understand the benefits of conflict resolution
  Understand intrapersonal conflict
  Understand interpersonal conflict
  Understand organizational conflict
  Understand drama triangle of victim, villain, and rescuer
  The courage to tell someone how they can do something better

---

Registered nurses (RNs) are consistently rated as the most honest and ethical profession by gallop polls each year. Registered nurses (RNs) should respect their patients while maintaining their dignity and protecting their patient rights. This respect extends to oneself and colleagues.

Professional ethics are principles that govern behavior in the work environment (◘ Fig. 9.5). Like values, professional ethics guide how others should act in the professional environment.

■ **Fig. 9.5** Ethical principles
(► http://ethics.iit.edu/teaching/
professional-ethics)

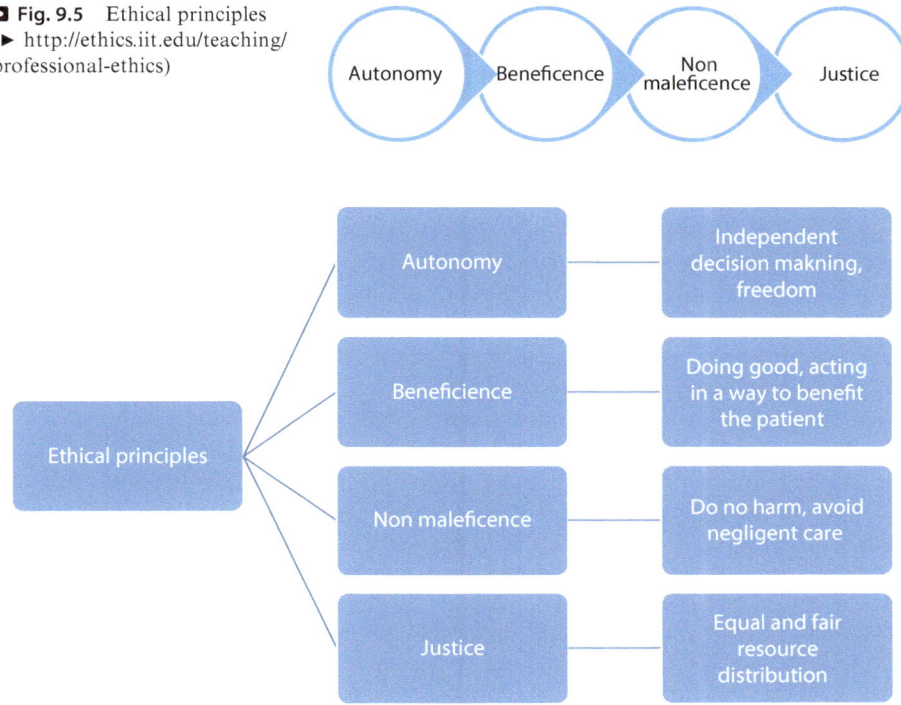

■ **Fig. 9.6** Four ethical principles with definitions

9.2.2 The ANA Code of Ethics with Interpretive Statements

The code of ethics for registered nurses (RNs) with interpretive statements by the ANA is an important tool for registered nurses (RNs) to use. The ANA includes statements about the wholeness of character, which describes the values of the nursing profession and one's moral values. Beauchamp and Childress (1979) described four principles of ethics which have gone on to become an essential foundation of analysis and resolution of bioethical problems. The four ethical principles include autonomy, beneficence, nonmaleficence, and justice (■ Fig. 9.6).

Autonomy involves the ability to self-rule and generates independent personal decisions. In nursing, respect for patient autonomy in situations such as obtaining informed consent for a procedure, treatment option, and disclosure of medical information is situational examples where patient autonomy may be addressed. Beneficence addresses the nurse's actions to benefit patients and ensure they're well-being. In nursing, an act believed to support a patient's "own good" is a way of supporting beneficence. For example, when a nurse encourages a patient to sit up for the first time after a procedure and stand, even though the patient hurts and complains, the nurse is demonstrating beneficence as this act is believed to support the patients well-being on their path to healing. Nonmaleficence is paired with beneficence and refers to "no harm." Nonmaleficence may involve making decisions to withhold treatment as a means to avoid negligent care by a nurse. Justice is a virtue-based concept and refers to the fair distribution of benefits and burdens in society. In nursing, justice may refer to scarce resources and the allocation of equitable distribution of the resources. For example, the determination of who has a right to healthcare and pay for the cost of healthcare.

The ANA code of ethics was first adopted in 1950. It is updated regularly to reflect changes in healthcare. The code supports registered nurses (RNs) in providing respective, humane, and dignified care to patients. While many registered nurses (RNs) possess these values, their ethics are challenged daily in the complex healthcare environment where care is not equitably distributed nor fair to all patients. There are nine provisions which make up the code, and they are divided into three major areas (◘ Fig. 9.7):

- Fundamental values and commitments of the registered nurse (RN)
- Boundaries of duty and loyalty to the profession of nursing
- Responsibilities of the registered nurse (RN) that extend beyond individual patient interactions

Together they provide statements of ethical values and dues of all registered nurses (RNs) and nursing students. The ethical standards are viewed as non-negotiable and clearly express the registered nurse (RN)'s commitment to society.

9.2.3 The ICN Code of Ethics for Nurses

The international council of nurses (ICN) adopted a code of ethics in 1953. The most current edition was updated in 2006. There are four principal elements in the ICN code that define nursing values: nurses and people, nurses and practice, nurses and profession, and nurses and coworkers (◘ Fig. 9.8). The nurses and people element describes the respect of patient values, spiritual beliefs, dignity, confidentiality, and customs. The nurses and practice element refer to the competency, accountability, and continued learning of professional conduct standards. The nurses and the profession element relate to advocacy, licensing, maintaining professional competence, and professional standards. The nurses and coworkers element refers to the cooperation and collaborative work in the nursing profession.

9.2.4 Ethical Dilemmas

Ethical dilemmas are prevalent in nursing practice. Nurses make ethical decisions on a daily basis and are typically not aware of the many ethical decision they make every day. An ethical dilemma is a situation where an individual must choose

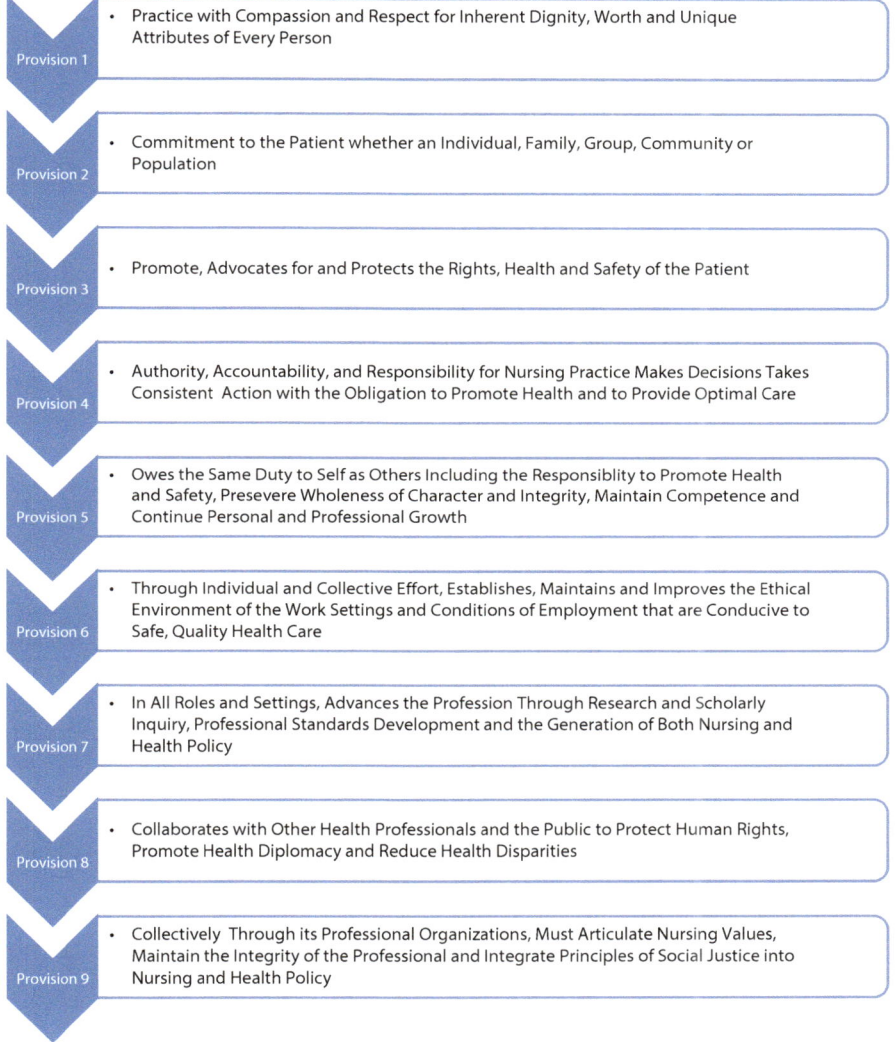

Provision 1
- Practice with Compassion and Respect for Inherent Dignity, Worth and Unique Attributes of Every Person

Provision 2
- Commitment to the Patient whether an Individual, Family, Group, Community or Population

Provision 3
- Promote, Advocates for and Protects the Rights, Health and Safety of the Patient

Provision 4
- Authority, Accountability, and Responsibility for Nursing Practice Makes Decisions Takes Consistent Action with the Obligation to Promote Health and to Provide Optimal Care

Provision 5
- Owes the Same Duty to Self as Others Including the Responsiblity to Promote Health and Safety, Presevere Wholeness of Character and Integrity, Maintain Competence and Continue Personal and Professional Growth

Provision 6
- Through Individual and Collective Effort, Establishes, Maintains and Improves the Ethical Environment of the Work Settings and Conditions of Employment that are Conducive to Safe, Quality Health Care

Provision 7
- In All Roles and Settings, Advances the Profession Through Research and Scholarly Inquiry, Professional Standards Development and the Generation of Both Nursing and Health Policy

Provision 8
- Collaborates with Other Health Professionals and the Public to Protect Human Rights, Promote Health Diplomacy and Reduce Health Disparities

Provision 9
- Collectively Through its Professional Organizations, Must Articulate Nursing Values, Maintain the Integrity of the Professional and Integrate Principles of Social Justice into Nursing and Health Policy

■ **Fig. 9.7** ANA ethical standards (▶ https://www.nursingworld.org/practice-policy/nursing-excellence/ethics/)

between two actions that may affect the well-being. Both actions can be justified as being good. One action must be chosen. For example, a nurse may be asked to work an extra shift during the workweek. The nurse may be tired and want to rest but is faced with the belief that choosing to work the extra shift will ensure safe care for the patients.

◻ Fig. 9.8   Four elements of
ICN code of ethics for nurses

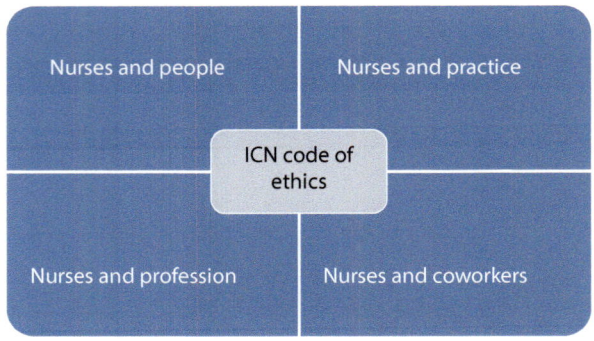

9.2.5 Moral Suffering

Moral suffering is experienced in nursing and is referred to as the disquieting feelings of anguish or uneasiness experienced when nurses sort out their emotions. They may realize situations that are morally unsatisfactory where forces are beyond their control result in moral suffering. The nurse may begin to believe the circumstances must be changed to ensure well-being to themselves or others. For example, when a doctor's order is not believed to be in the patient's best interest or the observation of perceived poor treatment by a family to a patient. Another example is the handling of an observed medical error by another nurse and the decision to report.

In any ethical situation, nurses must ask themselves, "what is good in terms of what one must do?" and "what is good in terms of how one wants to be?". Nurses must cultivate ethical behavior and habits and navigate through ethical dilemmas. Moral suffering cannot be eliminated or ignored in nursing. Through skills in decision-making, nurses can alleviate some of the effects of moral distress in nursing practice.

Each of these provisions can be applied and are applicable in many situations. When building your nursing career, understanding and knowledge of these provisions can guide decision-making.

9.3 Social Media

Social media includes websites and applications (apps) that allow users to participate in social networking, create, or share online content. On use of social media is to keep in touch with others, such as friends, extended family, or create new connections. People can connect on a global scale based on similar interests, feelings, insights, and emotions. Like other professions, the impact of social media on nursing has been significant. Social media benefits the profession by facilitating collaboration, the enhancement ideas on health issues, promotion of nursing, and improving overall population health. ▶ Case Example 9.3 describes six social networking principles described by the American Nurses Association (ANA).

1. Registered nurses (RNs) must not transmit or place online individually identifiable patient information
2. Registered nurses (RNs) must observe ethically prescribed professional patient-registered nurse (RN) boundaries
3. Registered nurses (RNs) should understand that patients, colleagues, organizations, and employers may view postings
4. Registered nurses (RNs) should take advantage of privacy settings and seek to separate personal and professional information online
5. Registered nurses (RNs) should bring the content that could harm a patient's privacy, rights, or welfare to the attention of appropriate authorities
6. Registered nurses (RNs) should participate in developing organizational policies governing online conduct

Typically, the principles seem like common sense. Unfortunately, issues still arise. Some tips to ensure you do not run into any problems are:

- Remember that standards of professionalism are the same online as in any other circumstance.
- Do not share or post information or photos gained through the registered nurse (RN)–patient relationship.
- Maintain professional boundaries in the use of electronic media. Online contact with patients blurs this boundary.
- Do not make disparaging remarks about patients, employers, or coworkers, even if they are not identified.
- Do not take photos or videos of patients on personal devices, including cell phones.
- Promptly report a breach of confidentiality or privacy.

There are both positive and negative impacts of social media.

9.3.1 Positive Aspects of Social Media

The public value of nursing is clear, and when the public is asked to defend nurses, they often cite anecdotal stories of personal experience with a nurse. The impact of nursing on society is positive. Nurses must understand their public image is the role of all nurses. The media plays a strong part in the societal view of professional nursing. Many views have been commonly advertised and stereotyped. For example, nurses are often portrayed as female.

Buresh and Gordan (2013) described actions for nurses to promote the real image in our profession. The hidden work of the nurse should be described and given a voice. Nurses should take opportunities to promote the profession through news, television, boards, legislation, etc. ▶ Case Example 9.4 includes a list of activities nurses can do to promote the image of the nursing profession.

Case Example 9.4 Actions for Nurses to Promote the Professional Nursing Image

Actions for nurses to promote the professional nursing image
  Educate the public in daily life
  Describe the nurses work
  Make known the "independent thinker" of the RN
  Deal with the fear of angering the medical doctor
  Accept thanks
  Take advantage of openings to promote nursing
  Respond to questions with real-life nursing stories
  Tell the details of nursing work
  Avoid nursing jargon
  Prepare to tell your story
  Do not suppress enthusiasm for nursing
  Reflect on nurses clinical judgment and competency
  Connect nursing work to pressing modern issues
  Respect patient confidentiality
  Resist with the fear of failure

9

9.3.2 Diversity in Nursing

Campaigns to promote diversity in nursing have recently been portrayed. For example, Johnson & Johnson continues to campaign a nursing future that supports public awareness of professional nursing. This positive promotion has supported recruitment into the profession. While a variety of opportunities for both women and men in nursing is shared, the disparity in a large number of women in the field remains. The increase in the number of men joining the nursing field has been significant, with an increase in the past several decades (◐ Fig. 9.9). In 1960, the number of men in nursing was 2.2%; in 2015, the percent of men in nursing has risen to 9%.

Similarly, there has been increasing diversity in race-ethnicity groups in nursing (◐ Fig. 9.10). This growth does not to match the growing diversity of the national population. For example, in 2014, ethnic and racial minority groups accounted for more than 38% of the US population. In 2017, 19% of the RN workforce represented minority backgrounds (AACN 2020). There is hope as the reported percentage of nursing students from minority backgrounds is 34%. The success of nursing in meeting the population healthcare needs requires a nursing workforce that matches the population served.

From a positive perspective, there is an ever-growing scope of social networking for registered nurses (RNs) seeking to build their careers. This technology has found its way into our everyday lives. Social media can be used to develop your career in many ways. One strategy is to choose a platform. LinkedIn is one of the most powerful career sites. Another strategy is to clean up your images on your personal sites. Consider if what you are posting puts your career in the best light. Remove anything that can offend or be considered in bad taste.

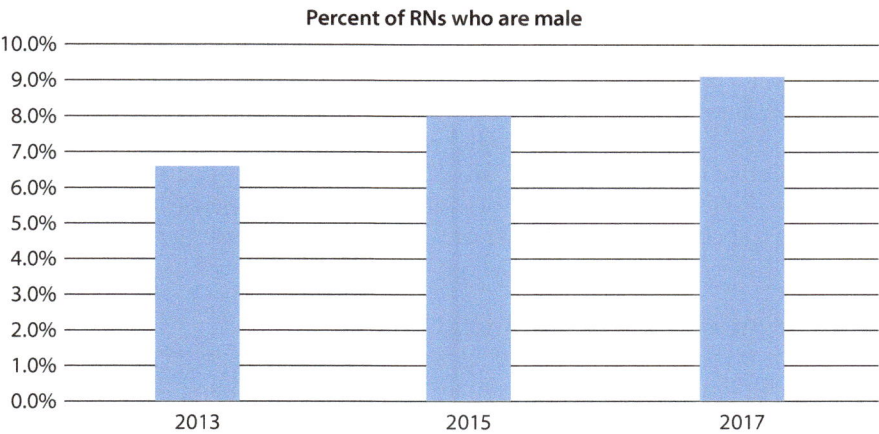

□ Fig. 9.9 Percentage of RNs who are male (► https://www.ncsbn.org/2018SciSymp_Smiley-Bienemy.pdf)

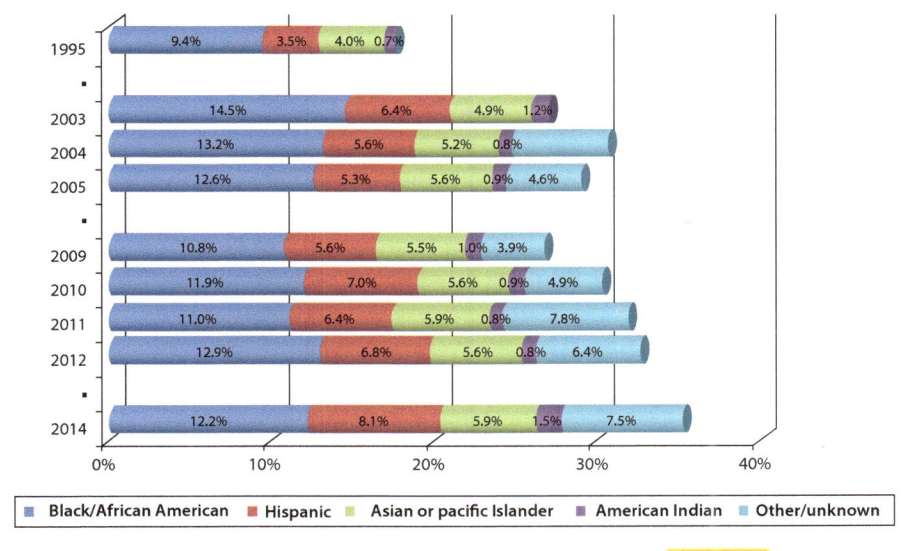

NLN Biennial Survey of Schools of Nursing, 2014

□ Fig. 9.10 Percent of minorities enrolled in basic RN programs by race-ethnicity (► http://www.nln.org/newsroom/nursing-education-statistics/nursing-student-demographics)

Connect with leaders in your field. Use keywords to connect with them. Also, connect with those at your level or below. Offer advice to those you can support. This behavior demonstrates your leadership skills. Connect with companies you admire. Get into a group with like-minded people.

Some may want to promote their own content. It is important to keep your message simple, use concepts that are easy to understand, and images that draw people in. Registered nurses (RNs) must effectively manage associated risks. Understand social media is for all to see. Use common sense.

9.3.3 Negative Aspects of Social Media

The negative impacts of social media are real. Registered nurses (RNs) have been sanctioned by boards of nursing for posting inappropriate and unethical pictures. Registered nurses (RNs) have lost their job for putting statements against others in the workplace or imposing their personal beliefs, which violate the ethical code for nursing.

There is a risk when coworkers communicate with each other using social media. This can be especially concerning when the communication is during work hours.

Key Questions to ask yourself:

- Does the content have the potential to damage a career or impair working relationships?
- Will the content breach your patient's trust or be detrimental to your employer?
- Will this harm others or me?

Social media can be an asset or hindrance to building your nursing career. Be careful in your use of it. When in doubt, do not post or comment until you are sure. Be sure you are familiar with your organization's policies and the guidelines described by the ANA. Once it is out there, it is difficult, if not impossible, to permanently remove unwanted information (► https://www.ncbi.nlm.nih.gov/pmc/articles/PMC2891246/).

9.4 Executive Presence

Some have called it the "it" factor. It is an executive presence. Think about a meeting when someone was speaking. Ask yourself, "did they attract and engage everyone?" Those with good executive presence are not "flustered." Executive presence is developed through self-awareness, reflection, and practice. Seven traits have been associated with a strong executive presence. There are several traits associated with a strong executive presence: composure, connection, confidence, credibility, clarity, conciseness, character, substance, and style. The last three in this list, character, substance, and style, make up the Bates Model of Executive Presence (◨ Fig. 9.11).

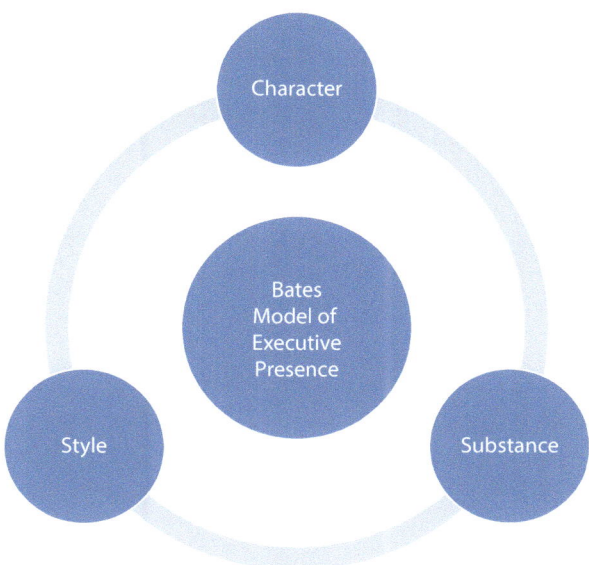

◘ Fig. 9.11 Bates model of executive presence (▶ https://www.bates-communications.com/what-we-do/assessments-expi/the-bates-model-of-executive-presence)

Composure This is a self-awareness and understanding that others are an essential component of executive presence. Composure is the ability to control your emotions and recognize emotion in others and manage your response to them.

Connection When communicating with others, the connection is essential to make them feel comfortable. Connecting is best achieved by understanding your communication style challenges and working on strategies to overcome them. Another essential component is improving your ability to read and adapt to the style of others. Registered nurses (RNs) have an ethical obligation to become skilled communicators as a component of their nursing practice.

Confidence Confidence must be communicated verbally and with body language. It starts with good posture. Eye contact is critical. You must speak by making eye contact and manage this communication appropriately with multiple people. Ensure your facial expression matches your message. Also, your voice should have a good pitch, volume, and pace. Your dress should be appropriate and carefully chosen. Before you walk into a meeting, take a minute to compose yourself, take a deep breath, and slow down. Always take time to prepare and consider what questions may be asked of you. If you are asked a question you cannot answer, do not doubt, "I don't know." Answer as best you can in a calm, collected manner.

Credibility Avoid using filler language such as "um," "uh," "so," which detracts from executive presence. Minimize "just," "sort of," and "this may not be a good idea…" When one with executive presence speaks, others notice and don't doubt the conviction in their words.

Clarity   Clear communication is essential. Points must be made clear, so attention from others is not lost. Ponder whether a message can be conveyed in 10 or fewer words. Ensure you can articulate it to yourself before communicating with others.

Conciseness   Being too wordy damages presence. Know what you want to communicate and do so in a concise way. Follow up by asking if you can share more information about this idea. This will ensure you can stay on point and expand the topic as needed for the listener (▶ https://www.businessinsider.com/the-7-traits-of-executive-presence-2013-9).

9.4.1 Character

Character is the core of a person. Their character is foundational and not observable. It is made of personal values as well as foundational characteristics such as courage, optimism, integrity, discretion, and priorities.

9.4.2 Substance

Substance includes traits that are cultivated over time. They include wisdom, confidence, and composure. These traits bring one's character and virtues together.

9.4.3 Style

Style is the most overt of the three. It is typically noted upon first impression and interpersonal behavior. The style must be congruent with the organization. Style often guides perception by others and can influence their opinion of the underlying substance.

Assessment tools are available to evaluate one's executive presences: ▶ https://www.bates-communications.com/what-we-do/assessments-expi/the-bates-model-of-executive-presence.

> **Strategies**
> Complete these free online quizzes:
>   What is your style of behavior? Use this online quiz to assess:
>   A Professional Behavior Quiz: ▶ https://www.proprofs.com/quiz-school/story.php?title=professional-behavior-quiz
>   A Professional Behavior in the Workplace Quiz: ▶ https://www.proprofs.com/quiz-school/story.php?title=professional-behavior-in-the-workplacecommunication-interpersonal-skills-34

Test your ethical behavior?

Integrity and Work Ethics Test: ► https://www.psychologytoday.com/us/tests/career/integrity-and-work-ethics-test

Quiz to determine if you have executive presence?

► https://redshoemovement.com/executive-presence-quiz/

Activities

In your next meeting, observe those around you. Who looks shy and unconfident? Who looks closed off? Are you sitting in a power stance? With your head looking forward, sitting tall, arms on the table, and not huddling within yourself. Are you maintaining eye contact with everyone in the room? When you speak, are you clear, firm, and loud enough to be heard? Do you end a sentence with purpose, not trailing off? Do you make those around you feel they are the only ones in the room? Do you really listen to others? Do you avoid speaking over others? Do you lean towards the person you are talking to and nod when they speak? Do you ask good questions to show you pay attention? Body Language can be more profound than verbal language (► https://www.themuse.com/advice/the-it-factor-how-to-have-executive-presence-in-a-meeting).

Vignettes

Vignette 1

In my career, I have made a conscious decision to advance my nursing career. This doesn't mean my ethical values are set aside. There are many situations where I have been faced with a decision to "do what is right." A "right" doesn't mean I directly benefit on the surface, wherein fact I do benefit because my moral compass is comfortable and in the correct direction as I know I did the right thing. If I didn't feel comfortable in my ethical decision-making, I am not sure I would like the person I see in the mirror every day.

Vignette 2

How do you handle a difficult patient?

I've often faced difficult patients. Handling them is part of the job. One patient, in particular, was yelling at everyone, even for minor problems. It was over a holiday, so I was able to get him moved to a private room. After that, I talked to him and realized he was upset over a hopeless diagnosis. He had no friends or family and nobody to talk to. I told the hospitalist, and she was able to get a therapist to speak with him. After that, he was actually pleasant. All the other staff and patients on the unit were visibly more relaxed. There's always a reason someone is difficult. Treating people with respect can often have surprising outcomes.

9.5 **Conclusions**

The path to building a successful nursing career is multifaceted and, indeed, a commitment. The process should begin with an assessment of oneself and what you stand for. Through this self-awareness journey, one can start to build a career that aligns with long- and short-term goals as well as with your values and beliefs. Goal setting is key as, without goals, you are on a journey with no direction. Once goals are identified, the path you follow may be one through advanced education or moving up the career ladder in your workplace, or both! Along the way, in order to be successful, you must grow within yourself but also support others through mentorship and role modeling.

The types of careers one can choose in registered nurses (RNs) are varied, and there is something for everyone. In addition to education and career ladder climbing, other strategies are needed. These include motivation, risk-taking, and ensuring a quality work/life balance. One must stay current and navigate in an ever-changing technology-driven world. Ongoing, lifelong professional growth is essential as this path of building a successful career is a journey, not a destination. Professional growth is a daily effort that includes professional development, an ongoing reflection of your developing strengths, and emerging weakness. Use your inward self-awareness to direct your growth initiatives. If you successfully use the strategies introduced in this book to guide the path to building your successful nursing career, you will find it will be rewarding and will feel less like a job and more like something you are passionate about, and you will never lose your drive to do better.

9.6 **Final Comments**

I would like to provide context to this book. The thoughts leading to the development of this book began many years back during my work with RN-BSN students working hard to advance their nursing careers. Once I move up in my organization, I realized this book was needed, and as soon as I felt the confidence to write it, I submitted my proposal to Springer. I was shocked; they accepted my proposal. My work began in mid-2019 and commenced in mid-2020. The COVID-19 pandemic developed during this time and impacted me personally and professionally as it did for nearly everyone worldwide. For anyone out there considering advancing their career or just possessing the thought, they want to embark on a professional journey in life; remember you are in the driver's seat. My work at my school of nursing was the most stressful it had ever been during the pandemic. We faced continuing the education and training of more than 1000 nursing students with dwindling opportunities for them to learn and study in hospital and community environments. In the end, life goes on, and in the word of my father-in-law who died in 2004, he told me, "Jenny, if you want to be a doctor in nursing, go for it. Don't worry about how old you will be. You will grow older anyway; the question is, will you be a doctor when you reach older age, or will you just still be thinking about becoming one?" I never forgot those words and missed his kindness and support.

References

American Association of Critical-Care Nurses (2020) Healthy Work Environment Standard. https://www.aacn.org/nursing-excellence/aacn-standards

Black (2016) Professional Nursing 8th Edition Elsevier

Beauchamp, T. L., & Childress, J. F. (1979) Principles of Biomedical Ethics. Oxford: Oxford University Press

Bostain, L. (2020). Nursing professionalism begins with you. American Nurse. June 25, 2020

Buresh, B. & Gordon, S. (2013) From Silence to Voice: What Nurses Know and Must Communicate to the Public. Cornell University Press

Callahan, D. & Jennings, B. (2002) Ethics and Public Health: Forging a Strong Relationship. American Journal of Public Health. 92(2):169–176

Fukada M (2018) Nursing competency: definition, structure and development. Yonago Acat Med 61(1):1–7. https://www.ncbi.nlm.nih.gov/pmc/articles/PMC5871720/

Hancock K (2020) Nursing and the journey to high reliability. https://consultqd.clevelandclinic.org/nursing-and-the-journey-to-high-reliability/

Pritchett, H. & Flexner, A. (2017) Medical Education in the United States and Canada: A Report to the Carnegie Foundation for the Advancement of Teaching. Andesite Press

Sortedahl C, Persinger S, Sobtzak K, Farrell B, Nicholas J (2017) Essential professional behaviors of nursing students and new nurses: hospital nurse leader perspectives survey. Nurs Educ Perspect 38(6):297–303. https://journals.lww.com/neponline/Abstract/2017/11000/Essential_Professional_Behaviors_of_Nursing.3.aspx